Nodira Husenova
Jakuthon Madzhidowa
Nargiza Jergasheva

EARLY DIAGNOSIS OF AUTISM SPECTRUM DISORDERS IN CHILDREN

Nodira Husenova
Jakuthon Madzhidowa
Nargiza Jergasheva

EARLY DIAGNOSIS OF AUTISM SPECTRUM DISORDERS IN CHILDREN

Results of the analysis of neuroprotein content and elemental composition of hair

Imprint

Any brand names and product names mentioned in this book are subject to trademark, brand or patent protection and are trademarks or registered trademarks of their respective holders. The use of brand names, product names, common names, trade names, product descriptions etc. even without a particular marking in this work is in no way to be construed to mean that such names may be regarded as unrestricted in respect of trademark and brand protection legislation and could thus be used by anyone.

Cover image: www.ingimage.com

This book is a translation from the original published under ISBN 978-620-7-64685-2.

Publisher:
Sciencia Scripts
is a trademark of
Dodo Books Indian Ocean Ltd. and OmniScriptum S.R.L publishing group

120 High Road, East Finchley, London, N2 9ED, United Kingdom
Str. Armeneasca 28/1, office 1, Chisinau MD-2012, Republic of Moldova, Europe
Printed at: see last page
ISBN: 978-620-7-62391-4

INTRODUCTION

In order to improve the effectiveness of measures to diagnose and treat autism, a wide range of scientific research is being conducted worldwide, aimed at studying the fundamental basis for the development of neurological complications, developing and improving diagnostic methods using modern methods of examination. Much attention is paid to studying the problems of early diagnosis of autism spectrum disorders; determining the causes of unsatisfactory treatment results; and improving prevention methods on the basis of modern research methods.

Many years of searching for a primary disorder, a suffering mental function responsible for the maladaptation of an autistic child, have not been successful, and currently, childhood autism is recognized as a pervasive, pervasive disorder of mental development. At present, the focus of attention of specialists is not so much on the manifestations of deficits in the individual mental abilities of an autistic child, but rather on the general patterns of developmental disorders in the forms of interaction with the surrounding world and, first and foremost, with a close person.

It is shown that progress in understanding the nature of childhood autism can be achieved only if we realize the unified logic of the disorder of the child's affective and cognitive development. Understanding that the formation of this type of mental dysontogenesis is associated with such profound violations of the organization of the child's relations with the world, brings to the forefront research focused on the earliest age. However, a number of important aspects of the early mental development of children with autism still remain insufficiently studied.

Development of means of early detection of tendencies of distortion of psychoneurological development and corrective support of the child before the final formation of the syndrome of infantile autism are aimed at improving the prognosis of his social adaptation.

CHAPTER I. CURRENT PROBLEMS OF DIAGNOSTICS AND TREATMENT OF AUTISM SPECTRUM DISORDERS IN CHILDREN

1.1 Autism spectrum disorders in children: a contemporary view of the problem

Autism spectrum disorders (ASD) are heterogeneous neurodevelopmental disorders that begin in early childhood and are characterized by deficits in social interaction and restricted patterns of repetitive/stereotyped behavior. Associated symptoms such as hyperactivity, irritability, insomnia, seizures, gastrointestinal and immune system dysfunction may occur

The concept of ASD was formed from the point of view of neuropsychiatric dysontogenesis, i.e. impaired development of such functions as emotions, perception, thinking, etc. However, over the past decades, a lot of evidence has accumulated that autism is not only a psychological disorder, as a certain part of children with RAS are diagnosed with genetic and chromosomal syndromes, various brain anomalies, metabolic diseases, etc. For a long time, the combination of autism with other clinical syndromes was not given special importance, but the high frequency of such cases eventually led to the emergence of the term "syndromal or atypical" autism, that is, when autism is one of the syndromes of another disease.

According to the ICD-10 International Classification of Diseases, autistic disorders proper include:

- Infantile autism (F84.0) (autistic disorder, infantile autism, infantile psychosis, Kanner syndrome);

- atypical autism (with onset after 3 years of age) (F84.1);

- Rett syndrome (F84.2);

- Asperger's syndrome - autistic psychopathy (F84.5);

The problem of autism in the world is beginning to take its toll in many ways and, above all, the number of people affected is increasing compared to previous years. According to WHO, the prevalence of autism is increasing by 14% every year and in China up to 20% per year. It is believed that the upward trend will continue in the future.

The etiology of RAS is quite complex. Genetic, epigenetic, infectious, autoimmune, metabolic, nutritional, and toxic factors may be involved. Various brain regions, neural pathways, neurotransmitters, neuropeptides, cytokines, synaptic molecules, and signal transduction processes may be affected (1). The etiology of autism can be identified in about 40% of cases, the cause of the rest is unknown (2). According to some authors, the risk of autism increases with increasing age of the father at the time of conception (3, 4, 5).

Chromosomal and genetic causes of autism may account for up to 50% of all cases of ASD, and the more severe the autism, the more likely its genetic origin (6, 7). In particular, autism affects up to 47% of patients with X-fragile chromosome syndrome, up to 10% of patients with Down syndrome, and up to 48% of patients with tuberous sclerosis (9).

In identical twins, ASD recurs in 70-97% of cases, and in dizygotic twins in 10-24%. An interesting fact is that one or another trait of autism is present in relatives of the patient in 90% of cases (8, 10). According to various scientists who have conducted most population studies, the prevalence of ASD is 1 per 100 girls and 4 per 100 boys (95).

Until recently, autism spectrum disorders were thought to be disorders of neurotransmitter metabolism, particularly serotonin. The following major hypotheses of autism are currently being considered:

1.	Increased excitability of the brain as a result of disturbance of the ratio of excitation and inhibition processes in nerve synapses (11)

2.   Abnormal development of the neuron itself and, as a result, abnormal synapse formation (12).

But in both cases, the unifying factor is the currently dominant cortical-disconnective model of autism (14), according to which ASD arises due to increased or decreased activity of functional connections and neuronal synchronization of neural pathways. This activity has been shown to correlate significantly with communicative, social, cognitive, and sensorimotor impairments in children with autism.

Increased excitability of brain neurons may serve as a pathogenetic basis for the development of epilepsy in patients with ASD. According to recent studies, the incidence of epilepsy in autism may be as high as 30% (13, 15). Epilepsy is more often observed in patients with moderate or severe forms of autism and has a very unfavorable effect on cognitive and emotional status.

Because of these complexities, the development of pharmacotherapy for ASD has progressed with great difficulty. The marked heterogeneity of these disorders suggests that different treatments will be effective for different patients. Early detection and intervention is needed when the brain is more plastic and changes are more easily reversible; however, some studies suggest that pharmacotherapy may also be effective in adults. Biomarkers can help stratify subgroups and predict response to treatment. The ultimate goal is to target nuclear symptoms of RAS; however, most current pharmacotherapeutic approaches target RAS-associated symptoms.

The atypical antipsychotics risperidone and aripiprazole are approved in the United States for the treatment of behavioral disorders (aggression, self-harm, angry outbursts) in children with ASD. The use of selective serotonin reuptake inhibitors (SSRIs), such as fluoxetine and citalopram, has been studied in the treatment of RAS: monocenter studies have shown their efficacy in affecting stereotypic behavior in children and adults, but multicenter studies have not demonstrated this efficacy, except in a group of subjects with increased irritability. The use of anticonvulsants has been studied for behavioral disorders such as impulsivity, self-injurious behavior, and aggression, which are common in RAS: valproates, acting through potentiation of inhibitory activity of the GABAergic system and through epigenetic effects, have shown efficacy in reducing irritability and impulsive-aggressive behavior in children with RAS. Drugs approved for the treatment of attention deficit hyperactivity disorder (ADHD) have also been used in studies for the treatment of children with ASD, and have shown moderate efficacy for symptoms such as hyperactivity (methylphenidate, dextraamphetamine, atomoxetine) and irritability (clonidine).

Newer experimental pharmacotherapeutic approaches to the treatment of RAS are based on knowledge of the molecular neurobiology and genetics of RAS (16). The action of one group of such drugs is aimed at preserving the balance of excitation and inhibition in cortical areas of the brain. These include targeting metabotropic glutamate receptors (such as mGlu5 antagonists), NMDA receptors (such as the NMDA receptor antagonist memantine), and AMPA receptors (such as the AMPA receptor potentiating drugs, ampakines). The use of mGlu5 antagonists has been investigated in subjects with RAS associated with X-linked fragile X syndrome and has shown promise in this subgroup of patients. GABAergic agents such as the GABA-B receptor agonist, arbaclofen (STX209), have shown efficacy for irritability and social isolation in children with RAS.

The peptide hormone oxytocin plays an important role in social interaction and behavior. In adults with ASD, intravenous administration of high-dose oxytocin reduced stereotypic behavior and gradually improved the clarity of emotion recognition in speech. Administration intranasally improved social interaction in children, adolescents, and adults with RAS. A vasopressin receptor 1a antagonist had an effect on the recognition of emotions in speech, such as fear and passion, in adults with high-functioning RAS.

Insulin-like growth factor 1 (IGF-1) plays an important role in nervous system maturation, development, and connectivity, which is impaired in RAS. Studies in mice with a mutation in the Shank-3 gene, which is a model of Phelan-McDermid syndrome that may be associated with some cases of RAS, have shown that IGF-1 can reverse structural changes in ionotropic glutamate receptors, alterations in functional synaptic plasticity, and disturbances in excitation/inhibition balance. A clinical trial of recombinant human IGF-1 in children with Phelan-McDermid syndrome showed improvement in the areas of social isolation and restricted behavior.

Immunosuppressive drugs and protein synthesis inhibitors, such as the mTOR inhibitor rapamycin, have been shown to be effective for social isolation in some forms of RAS.

The alpha-7 nicotinic acetylcholine receptor (nACR) gene is associated with autism in ADHD. nACR drugs, including mecamylamine, transdermal nicotine administration, and donesepil, have been used in clinical trials. Some alpha-7 nACR antagonists, such as galantamine, have shown promise in animal models and clinical trials.

Complementary and alternative medicine have also been investigated in the therapy of RAS. However, they cannot be clearly regulated and have not been studied in large-scale clinical trials. Moreover, their safety and efficacy have not been precisely determined. Treatment with dietary supplements may complement, but not replace, approved treatments for RAS. Melatonin can be used for sleep disorders, omega-3 fatty acids for stereotypic behavior and improved socialization. Vitamin B12 preparations are hypothesized to protect against oxidative damage in RAS. Curcumin, the active ingredient in turmeric, may be beneficial in RAS, possibly due to its antioxidant and anti-inflammatory properties. Probiotics, such as yogurt, may have beneficial effects on the gut microbiome and on proinflammatory cytokines that may play a role in the pathogenesis of RAS.

As a result, the incredible heterogeneity of RAS complicates the development of new pharmacotherapies. Personalized treatment is preferred, and studies of populations with orphan diseases may accelerate the development of pharmacotherapies. The design of future clinical trials should focus on patient stratification based on biomarkers and etiology (e.g., immune-inflammatory) and target populations stratified by clinical symptoms.

New psychopharmacologic approaches such as oxytocin/vasopressin antagonists, anti-inflammatory agents, IGF-1, drugs that regulate excitation/inhibition processes, protein synthesis inhibitors, and microbiome-targeted drugs may definitely be promising. Existing medications such as anticonvulsants, SSRIs, and atypical antipsychotics may be effective in some patients. It is important to study the efficacy of medications in young children who may benefit from early intervention. The ultimate goal of RAS pharmacotherapy will be to link therapy to the molecular mechanisms underlying the disease in each patient.

1.2 The neuropathology of autism

RAS are characterized by dynamic age-dependent structural and functional abnormalities. Developmental heterochrony, in which different parts of the brain grow at different rates, is a defining anatomical feature associated with the disorder (Carper & Courchesne, 2016; Carper et al., 2016; Carper et al., 2015; Courchesne et al., 2011; Sparks et al., 2015). Topographic changes caused by developmental heterochrony are likely to result in changes in cytoarchitectonics that allow for the distinction of specific neurological disorders in autism. Further deviation from the normal trajectory of brain development may be used as a means of diagnosing specific subtypes in the future (Courchesne et al., 2014). Disorders of local and global connectivity are characterized by overdevelopment of local connectivity networks to the detriment of long-range connectivity (Casanova et al., 2013; Courchesne & Pierce, 2016). The following are developmental abnormalities typical of RAS. They are sources of structural and functional changes that form the clinical phenotype. Children with RAS typically have macrocephaly and macroencephaly, two features that are evident before and at the time of clinical diagnosis. Despite conflicting data, at least one long-term study has shown that head circumference in children with RAS is significantly smaller at birth than in neurotypical children (Courchesne et al., 2014), but becomes significantly larger by 6-14 months of age (Courchesne et al., 2014). Head circumference measures have suggested the exact size of the brain, and MRI studies, have shown that brain volume in autistic children is larger than in control children (Bartholomeusz et al., 2015; Piven et al., 2010). Brain volume in autistic children most often increases between 2 and 4.5 years of age, with cerebellar and cerebral white matter (CWM) being the main cause of the increase (Courchesne et al., 2011). This macroencephaly appears to be prone to manifest in certain areas, but the results of volumetric studies are conflicting. For example, one study showed that the increase in BV volume occurs more in the frontal lobes and less in the occipital lobes. However, other studies suggest that volume increases are more intrinsic to the occipital and parietal lobes (Filipek, 2010; Piven et al., 2010). Excessive brain growth may also be related to genetic polymorphisms of key neurotransmitters (Wassink et al., 2017; Davis et al., 2017; Razanahan et al., 2009). Acceleration of brain growth precedes and is associated with the onset of clinical symptoms, and specific growth patterns reflect the severity of RAS (Courchesne et al., 2014; Dawson et al., 2017; Dementieva et al., 2016).

Brain growth trajectories in children with ASD slow down after the first year of life, level off in adolescence, and are comparable to normal in adulthood (Redclay & Courchesne, 2016). The functional consequences of the abnormal brain development seen in autism explain many of the behavioral features characteristic of the disorder (Cohen, 2017). Although the brain size of autistic patients in adulthood is quite comparable to that of controls, the intrinsic pathology remains and shows that functional connectivity across domains is impaired.

MRI studies reveal many distinctive neuroanatomical features associated with autism, such as a significant increase in the volume of the BV. Typically, the BV occupies less than one-third of the total brain volume, but autistic patients have 65% more of it than controls (Herbert et al., 2014). With equal total brain volume, autistic patients demonstrate a higher volume of BV than controls of the same age. This suggests that increased BV volume is a feature associated with autism rather than a manifestation of macrocephaly (Bigler et al., 2010; Herbert et al., 2014). When the BV of the brain was divided into an outer zone consisting of interhemispheric cortico-cortical connections and an inner zone containing connective and sagittal compartments, an increase in outer BV was observed in all brain lobes with predominance in the frontal lobes, whereas no increase in inner BV was observed in autism (Herbert et al., 2015). Also, compared to controls, autism showed decreased BV volume in different regions of the corpus callosum (Hardan et al., 2017; Hardan et al., 2019; Piven et al., 2021).

As with the data on overall brain enlargement, the concentration of BV in older autistic patients is slightly higher than in controls (Chung et al., 2014; Waiter et al., 2015). Overgrowth of certain regions of the BV is part of a pathological process that disrupts the development of normal brain structure and function in autism, although the molecular mechanisms underlying these processes are currently not well understood. Volumetric analyses indicate that abnormalities in multiple cortical and subcortical structures are associated with autism. The limbic system, which is responsible for emotion, memory, and motivation, is invariably affected. The results of several studies suggest reduced size of the amygdala and hippocampus in autistic patients, as well as reduced performance on neuropsychological tasks involving these areas (Aylward et al., 2016; Herbert et al., 2014; Loveland et al., 2017; Saitoh et al., 2011). However, other studies show that the volume of the hippocampus of children with autism is larger compared to controls, and the amygdala is enlarged only in young children with autism (Schumann et al., 2015). While these parts of the limbic system may be larger in children with autism, they are smaller in adults compared to controls (Aylward et al., 2016). Optic nerve abnormalities have also been observed and include increased cell packing density, decreased cell size, and an overall decrease in optic nerve volume in patients with autism (Hardan et al., 2013; Schultz et al., 2016; Tsatsanis et al., 2014). Increased volume of the occipitotemporal lobe and cerebellar hemisphere is associated with autism (Brambilla et al., 2014). Excessive growth of the frontal and temporal lobes and the amygdala coincides with an abnormal increase in brain growth rate that occurs between 2 and 4 years of age in children with autism. Although cortical thinning usually occurs with age, the process is faster in patients with autism.

According to voxel-wise MRI, gray matter content is reduced in certain areas and total cerebrospinal fluid volume is significantly increased in patients with autism compared to controls. Other studies suggest an increase in gray matter volume in certain areas in autism (Rojas et al., 2013). Although some fMRI studies have produced conflicting results, they have found unbalanced brain growth in early childhood autism, in which growth trajectories are atypical and regionally differentiated. The first attempts to study neuropathologic changes in autism were made in the 1980s by many groups. As a result, five neuropathologic features were associated with autism: increased brain weight and BV volume in childhood, reduced neuronal size and increased cell packing density in the forebrain limbic system, decreased number of Purkinje cells in the brain, age-related changes in cell size and number of nuclei in the diagonal gyrus, cerebellum, and inferior olive, and malformations of the cortex and brainstem.

Postmortem studies of autism most often show a significant reduction in the number of Purkinje cells in the cerebellum compared to controls. The size of Purkinje cells in autism is also smaller compared to controls of the same sex and age. Abnormalities in the size and number of neurons in the blood, globular, and cork nuclei are also present and appear to change with age. What follows is a summary of the list of neuropathologic features of autism observed by the different groups.

Cortical and subcortical morphologic abnormalities associated with autism most commonly involve the limbic system.

Histologic studies have shown that autistic patients have smaller hippocampal cell size and simplified dendritic branching compared to controls of the same age (Raymond et al., 2010).

Data regarding the size and packing density of neurons in the amygdala in autism are inconsistent. While some studies show a decrease in neuronal size and an increase in packing density, others show no significant difference in cell size but a significant decrease in the number of neurons in the amygdala in autistic patients. According to the data, cell packing density in the hypothalamus and mastoid body is increased . Smaller neuronal size has been found in the basal ganglia and cerebellum in autistic children from 4 to 7 years of age, especially in Purkinje cells, dentate nuclei, amygdala, contiguous nucleus, caudate nucleus, and shell . As the adult grows older, the size comes to normal. A general decrease in the density of axons and dendrites in the autistic brain has also been observed . These studies indicate a stunted neuronal growth, as evidenced by cortical dysplasia, which is dependent on brain structure, occurs in autism and undergoes changes during life. Neuropathologic studies of autism have revealed several morphologic abnormalities of the brainstem and cerebellum. An abundance of neurons in the nuclei of the inferior olive is observed, but their size changes with age. Thus, they are larger in children younger than 12 years of age and smaller in adults older than 21 years of age than in controls of the same age . The areas of the varioli pontine, medulla oblongata, and mid-sagittal region are smaller in autistic patients, and the varioli pontine appears to develop more rapidly in autism than in controls. As mentioned earlier, the cerebellum is the most common site of abnormality in autism. Changes in Purkinje cell density and number are more prominent in certain areas . Hyperplasia and hypoplasia are noticeable in the cerebellar vermis region . These studies indicate the presence of atrophy of the cortex of the lateral parts of the cerebellar hemispheres and lack of Purkinje cells in some areas. It is possible that some of these changes are the result of agonal and preagonal changes.

Recent brain findings from the Autism Tissue Program (ATP) (n=35) showed that approximately one-third of the patients (n=11) died from drowning (two received cardiopulmonary resuscitation and remained alive indefinitely). The remaining twenty-three died of various causes including: hypoxia, seizures, circulatory failure, blood poisoning, anoxic encephalopathy, etc. Most likely, hypoxia or hypoxia together with reperfusion may have caused the loss of vulnerable cell types (e.g. Purkinje cells) or neuroinflammatory changes. In fact, some of the incidences of nerve inflammation (e.g., predominant white matter gliosis) in autistic patients are similar to those who died after asphyxiation or drowning. Therefore, these changes may reflect the cause of death of the patients rather than the autism pathology itself. Neocortical minicolumns, the basic architectonic and functional units of the human brain into which neurons in the cerebral cortex are grouped, are smaller, more numerous, and less compact in autistic patients than in controls.

Although this pathology was observed bilaterally in Brodmann's 3, 4, 9, 17, 21, and 22 fields, the narrowest minicolumns were found in the dorsolateral prefrontal cortex of the brains of autistic patients.

The decrease in the size of neocortical neurons and their nuclei is most likely an indicator of reduced or impaired functional connectivity between distant cortical areas with a tendency toward local rather than global information processing. Reduced size of the corpus callosum and gyrus confirms the presence of a restricted cortical network of connections that favors short-range cortico-cortical fibers over long-range commissural fibers.

Cortical malformations have been observed in disorders caused by abnormalities of cell proliferation, apoptosis,

cell migration, cortical organization, and axonal guidance. Thus, the minicolumn abnormalities found in autistic patients suggest that the cause of the initial pathology appears to lie during embryonic or early postnatal development.

Studies of clinicopathologic correlations in autism have found links between several areas of functional deficit and primary nervous system abnormalities. One of the main features of ASD symptomatology includes limited speech abilities related to understanding semantics and social pragmatics . Studies of areas of the neocortex responsible for speech have shown decreased neuronal density in Wernicke's area (PB 22) and angular gyrus (PB 39), and increased glial cell density in these areas and in Broca's area (PB 44) in autistic patients compared to controls. The researchers hypothesize that structural changes in cortical areas responsible for speech are responsible for the occurrence of communication disorders in autistic patients. Another important feature of RAS patients is impaired social interaction, eye contact and facial expressions. Autistic patients have been found to have problems with face recognition, perception and recognition. Studies using functional magnetic resonance imaging (fMRI) have shown in autistic patients reduced activity of the spindle gyrus, which is responsible for recognizing human facial features . This reduced activity is thought to be related to the inability of autistic patients to make direct eye contact.Neuropathological studies have found reduced number and volume of neurons in the spindle gyrus and have suggested that underdevelopment of connections between the primary visual cortex (PB 17) and the spindle gyrus is responsible for poor facial feature recognition in autism (van Kooten et al., 2017). Disorders of gross and fine motor skills are also very common in patients with autism . It is hypothesized that sensory-motor impairments may be associated with pathologic changes in the basal ganglia and cerebellum. A positive correlation between caudate nucleus volume and the frequency of such symptoms in autism has been observed. The cerebellar findings, which include decreased numbers of GABAergic Purkinje cells and increased direct inhibition via basket neurons, suggest altered cerebellar cell inhibition, which may have a direct effect on cerebellar and cortical sends and lead to changes in motor and perceptual performance . The defined range of cognitive impairment in autism shows that patients' nonverbal IQ is usually higher than verbal IQ, and that perceptual levels on intelligence tests are usually low.

These cognitive impairments are most likely related to disturbances in the memory and limbic systems. Reduced size of the hippocampal formation and amygdala in autism, as well as simplified dendritic branching in the hippocampus, have been observed. Reduced volume of the anterior cingulate gyrus and decreased brain activity on positron emission tomography (PET) scans have also been seen in autistic patients . The caudate nucleus is responsible for learning, short-term and long-term memory, planning, and problem solving, so observing changes in the caudate nucleus in autistic children may help explain the cognitive deficits characteristic of autism. Neuroanatomical and neuropathologic studies have revealed an atypical developmental pattern in ASD. The brains of autistic patients are usually larger at the onset of clinical symptoms than those of controls. The reason is a disproportionate increase in white matter volume in some areas. Heterochrony of development is one of the defining features of RAS, but discrepancies in the results make it impossible to cross-compare them. These discrepancies involve many factors, most notably conflicting patient diagnoses and exclusion criteria. A statistical challenge is the collection of data, due to the small sample size. The results are also skewed by factors such as comorbidities, IQ, time since death, cause of death, and medical history. However, despite the conflicting data it is clear that characteristic neurological disorders are associated with the core symptoms of RAS. Visual analysis can be used to identify individuals with autistic disorders, Asperger's syndrome, or pervasive developmental disorder and therefore may be widely used in diagnosis. Typical processing impairments associated with neuronal network limitations underlie the observed and defining behaviors in ASD and suggest that autism is a disorder related to neural information processing. How specifically these neurobiological disorders affect the behavioral phenotype is still under investigation. Summarizing all the data, it appears that although the abnormalities observed in the brains of autistic patients represent a long-term neuropathology that continues to change into adulthood, this process may have a prenatal origin.

1.3 Macro- and micronutrients in the etiology and pathogenesis of autism spectrum disorder in children

Attempts to find a relationship between elemental status and RAS in children, according to Pubmed data, were made back in the late 1970s– early 1980s (Gentile et al., 1983). Significant differences in the elemental status of children with RAS were reported: lower concentrations of calcium, magnesium, copper, manganese, chromium, cobalt and higher concentrations of lithium in hair compared to the normotypic population (Wecker et al., 1985).

Studies in the 2000s partially confirmed the findings of Wecker et al. For example, Al-Ayadhi found significantly lower concentrations of calcium, copper, chromium, manganese, iron, and cobalt in hair samples of children with ASD compared to normotypic children (Al-Ayadhi, 2016). Studies by Adams et al, as well as Skalny et al, reported nearly twofold lower iodine and chromium levels in the hair of children with RAS (Adams et al, 2013; Skalny et al, 2017).

Priya and Geetha (2011) demonstrated that the concentrations of magnesium and selenium in the hair and nails of children with ASD were significantly reduced compared to the control group. In addition, copper levels in the hair of children were shown to correlate with the severity of RAS manifestations. Low copper levels in hair were associated with high-functioning autism. The study also showed a significant decrease in zinc concentration in hair and nails in children from the low-functioning autism group compared to the control group (Priya, Geetha, 2011).

Yasuda et al. reported that magnesium and zinc deficiency in hair is characteristic of a group of young children with RAS (0– 3 years), and in older children it is almost leveled out (Yasuda et al., 2013).

Blaurock-Busch et al. found a negative correlation between zinc concentration in hair and manifestations of nervousness and phobia in children with RAS (Blaurock-Busch et al., 2012).

In contrast, in a study by Al-Farsi et al. children with RAS had significantly higher levels of elements such as sodium, magnesium, potassium, zinc and iron, but lower levels of calcium and copper in hair samples (Al-Farsi et al., 2013).

Low calcium levels in the hair of children with ASD were also reported by Blaurock-Busch et al. and Fiłon et al. (Blaurock-Busch et al., 2012; Fiłon et al., 2020). Meta-analysis is a sensitive method of analyzing a large number of original studies devoted to a specific problem and assessing the reliability of the results obtained.

A recent systematic review and meta-analysis by Saghazadeh et al. confirms the differences in the elemental status of hair of children with RAS compared to normotypic children. The study showed that hair chromium, cobalt, iodine, iron, and magnesium contents were significantly lower in patients with RAS than in control subjects.

The findings help to emphasize the role of elements in the development of RAS (Saghazadeh et al., 2017). All these studies conducted in different parts of the world suggest the presence of imbalances of vital minerals and altered heavy metal levels in the hair of children with RAS. Conflicting data on the content of individual elements in the hair of patients with RAS require further investigation to identify associated factors likely to influence the outcome - such as area of residence and geochemical features of the area, regional nutritional characteristics, genetic features of element metabolism, sex and age composition of the study groups, type of RAS, antagonistic interactions between elements, etc.

Magnesium is a regulatory cation that modulates gamma-aminobutyric acid (GABA) signaling and influences inhibition processes in the nervous system (Stangherlin et al., 2018). Recent work by Yamanaka et al. has shown that magnesium ions are required for activation of the CREB and mTOR signaling pathways (the CREB and mTOR signaling pathways) and contribute to the structural and functional maturation of neuronal networks. Magnesium ion release was mediated by GABAA receptor (GABAA receptor) activity (Yamanaka et al., 2018). In turn, an imbalance between the excitatory (glutamate-mediated) and inhibitory (GABAA-mediated) systems of the brain is a common pathophysiological mechanism in RAS (Coghlan, 2012). Excessive levels of glutamate and other excitatory molecules lead to overexcitation and activation of ionotropic glutamate receptors (NMDAR and AMPAR) with subsequent calcium cumulation in neurons and the occurrence of excitatory neurotransmitter toxicity (excitotoxicity, excitotoxicity) (Strunecka et al., 2018). Increased calcium levels in the cytosol are explained by the fact that excess glutamate leads to a longer opening of calcium channels and increased calcium influx into cells. The influx of intracellular calcium triggers the production of free radicals, which ultimately leads to mitochondrial dysfunction and cell apoptosis (Essa et al., 2013). Magnesium, on the other hand, through regulation of NMDAR activity, reduces intracellular calcium concentration and neuronal excitability (Blanke et al., 2009). Magnesium has also been shown to play a role in the regulation of neuroinflammatory response, which is another pathogenetic mechanism of RAS development. Magnesium modulates the activity of transcription factors such as nuclear factor kappa-bi (NF-kB). NF-κB is a protein present in almost all cell types and provides regulation of the immune response by inducing the expression of inflammatory cytokines and chemokines (Young et al., 2011). In recent work, magnesium has been shown to prevent NF-κB activation by inhibiting nuclear translocation and phosphorylation of NF-κB (Hu et al., 2018). Magnesium, along with multivitamins, probiotics, vitamin D3 and omega-3 fatty acid preparations, is among the most common complementary therapies for RAS. In a study by Trudeau et al. (2019), it was observed that 28.1% of the studied patients with RAS received magnesium preparations. However, the efficacy of these medications has not yet been confirmed (Trudeau et al., 2019). In particular, the 2013 Cochrane meta-analysis found insufficient evidence of the efficacy of MagnesiumB6 in the treatment of RAS (Nye, Brice, 2016).

Calcium plays a critical role in the development of the nervous system (Lohmann, 2009). Intracellular calcium acts as a secondary messenger and has many regulatory functions. It is well known that in nerve endings, calcium activates the release of neurotransmitters (Neher et al., 2017). Signal transduction is enabled by calcium-binding proteins that capture changes in cellular calcium ion concentration by interacting with downstream regulatory targets. One example of such calcium sensor proteins is the family of neuronal calcium sensors (NCSs), which are expressed predominantly in neurons and photoreceptor cells (Weiss et al., 2010). Neuronal calcium receptor-1 (NCS-1) is involved in neurotransmission, axon outgrowth, synaptic plasticity, learning and motivated behavior (Dason et al., 2012). A study by deRezende et al. in a mouse model showed that lack of NCS-1 leads to depressive and anxious behavior, impairments in spatial reasoning and memory (de Rezende et al., 2014). Disruptions in NCS-1 are found in a number of neuropsychiatric conditions such as schizophrenia, bipolar disorder (D'Onofrio et al., 2014) and RA (Piton et al., 2017). Other known calcium sensors– extracellular calcium-sensitive receptors (CASRs), which regulate parathyroid glands and systemic calcium homeostasis, are also present in neurons and help control axonal and dendritic growth in the developing brain (Vizard et al., 2017). Liu et al. in an animal model study demonstrated the role of CASRs in the formation of interneuronal connections and myelination. Mice with CASR receptors turned off (a model of neonatal hyperparathyroidism) had reduced brain weight and showed delayed proliferating cell nuclear antigen expression (Liu et al., 2013). Calcium channelopathies are associated with various neuropsychiatric diseases such as schizophrenia, manic depressive psychosis, migraine, and RAS (Gargus 2009; Berridge, 2014). In a recent Genome-wide association study, it was shown that impaired calcium signaling is a common pathogenetic factor for these psychopathological conditions (Cross-Disorder Group of the Psychiatric Genomics Consortium, 2013).

Potassium and sodium channels are highly heterogeneous proteins that are widely expressed in the CNS, where they set the membrane resting potential of neurons and glia, form the action potential, regulate the conduction of nerve impulses, activation and release of neurotransmitters. Their dysfunction is a major contributor to nervous system dysfunction (Eijelkamp et al., 2012) and leads to the appearance of impaired social behavior (Bausch et al., 2018). A growing number of studies suggest a role for genetic defects in ion channels (channelopathies) in the pathogenesis of RAS. Canalopathies have profound effects on brain function by disrupting extra- and intracellular macronutrient homeostasis (Schmunk et al., 2013). In recent years, high-throughput sequencing capabilities have identified polymorphisms and rare variants in genes regulating calcium, sodium, and potassium channels that predispose to RAS (Weiss et al., 2014; Lee et al., 2014), as well as associated disorders such as epilepsy (Keller et al., 2017), ADHD (Rejersen et al., 2017), and migraine (Gargus, 2009). Interestingly, patients with RAS who have potassium or sodium channelopathy are more likely to suffer from concomitant epilepsy as well (D'Adamo et al., 2011a).

Zinc plays an important role in neurogenesis by regulating the rate of DNA, RNA, and protein synthesis in the brain, neuronal migration, neurotransmission in the hippocampus, and insulin-like growth factor-1 (IGF-1) gene expression (Adamo et al., 2010). Sufficient zinc intrauterine is important for proper development and function of the hippocampus, cerebellum, and autonomic nervous system (Fuglestad et al., 2017). Zinc ensures the production of metallothioneins (Park et al., 2011), which are necessary for the detoxification of heavy metals in the body (Aschner, 2010). Coghlan et al. (2012) suggested that dysfunction in excitatory and inhibitory synapses is responsible for RAS symptoms and that micronutrients in particular mediate synaptic function (Coghlan et al., 2012). A recent study showed that zinc deficiency interferes with excitatory synaptic activity, resulting in behavioral abnormalities characteristic of RAS (Grabrucker et al., 2014). Low zinc levels are also associated with the development of depression (Swardfager et al., 2013), attention deficit hyperactivity disorder (Lepping et al., 2010), and epilepsy (Saghazadeh et al., 2015).

Copper is also actively involved in synaptic transmission (Grabrucker et al., 2014; Opazo et al., 2014). Altered copper levels, in particular, have a direct effect on monoaminergic transmission systems by reducing norepinephrine and dopamine levels (Santos et al., 2019). Copper imbalance can disrupt the metabolic balance between the body's antioxidant systems and free radicals (reactive oxygen species), triggering oxidative stress processes. Increased free radical levels contribute, in turn, to cellular oxidative damage, impaired antioxidant defenses in the body, changes in immune response, and thus neuroinflammation (Santos et al., 2019).

Oxidative stress has long been known as a mechanism underlying numerous diseases and their associated complications, particularly neurodegenerative diseases, diabetes mellitus and cancer (Reuter et al., 2010). Disruption of copper homeostasis in the intrauterine period can increase the risk of RAS (Li et al., 2014) and inevitably leads to alterations in cognitive and motor development (Santos et al., 2019). In addition, copper serves as a cofactor for a number of enzymes involved in various metabolic functions and redox reactions: superoxide dismutase 1 and 3 (SOD1 and SOD3) for antioxidant activity, cytochrome-C oxidase for ATP production in mitochondria, lysyl oxidase for collagen maturation, tyrosinase for melanin synthesis, ceruloplasmin (CP) for iron metabolism, etc.п. (Spain et al., 2009; Fukaj et al., 2011; Solano, 2018; Vallet et al., 2019).

The central nervous system is the most susceptible to thyroid hormone levels (Prezioso et al., 2018). Their deficiency during critical periods of brain development, both in utero and in the early postnatal period, is a recognized cause of irreversible brain damage leading to mental retardation, reduced intellectual ability (up to cretinism), psychomotor retardation and deafness. Prior to intrauterine thyroid formation (between the 12th and 17th week of gestation), the fetus is unable to produce free thyroxine (FT4) and is completely dependent on maternal FT4, which penetrates the blood-brain barrier. Reduced maternal FT4 levels can have a negative impact on fetal development (Román, 2017). Román also hypothesized that maternal hypothyroxinemia during pregnancy may contribute to the development of autism (Román, 2017). Moreover, more than half of children with ASD and their mothers are iodine deficient (Hamza etal., 2013). A 2015 cohort study reported a higher prevalence of elevated maternal thyroperoxidase antibodies in cases of autism in their children (Brown et al., 2015). In another cohort study, maternal thyroid dysfunction in early pregnancy was associated with the development of epilepsy, RAS and ADHD in the child (Andersen et al., 2018). A study by Levie et al. found that low maternal free thyroxine (FT4) was associated with lower IQ in their children. Hypothyroxinemia was also found to be associated with a high risk of autistic traits (Levie et al., 2018). Another study by the same author did not confirm the association of maternal iodine deficiency and the occurrence of autistic traits in children (Levie et al., 2020). The work of Błażewicz et al. reported an association between autism symptoms and reduced urinary iodine excretion in boys with RAS (Błażewicz et al., 2016). A study by Tinkov et al. showed an association between low hair iodine levels in RAS patients and catatonic syndrome (Tinkov et al., 2018). However, there is currently no conclusive evidence for the causal significance of an altered thyroid profile and RAS (Andersen et al., 2018).

Decreased iron concentration in the brain is accompanied by changes in the serotoninergic and dopaminergic systems, leads to impaired conduction of cortical fibers and myelogenesis in general (Erikson et al., 2011). Perinatal iron deficiency has a significant impact on learning and memory, information processing speed and socioemotional regulation (Lozoff et al., 2013). A direct correlation between ferritin levels and impaired communication has been reported (Dosman et al., 2013). Iron deficiency has been described in a whole spectrum of neuropsychiatric problems such as delayed psycho-speech development, emotional-verbal and behavioral disorders in children, and cognitive deficits (Mccann, Ames, 2017; Lozoff et al., 2017). Evidence suggests impaired iron homeostasis in neurodegenerative diseases (Benarroch, 2009), depression, and anxiety (Lozoff et al., 2017). Researchers have reported a high prevalence of iron deficiency in children with RAS. For example, a study by Hergüner et al. found that 24.1% of children with RAS had latent iron deficiency and 15.5% had iron deficiency anemia– (Hergüner et al., 2012).

The effect of selenium on brain function is mainly mediated by its involvement in the activity of selenoproteins - glutathione peroxidases

(GPXs), thioredoxin reductases (TXNRDs), selenoprotein P (SELENOP) and methionine sulfoxide reductase B (MSRB). Mechanisms for the putative neuroprotective effects of selenium in RAS may include inhibition of oxidative stress and suppression of the neuroinflammatory response. Selenium reduces oxidative stress by modulating antioxidant activity and cytosolic Ca2+ influx into nerve cells (Skalny et al., 2018). In addition to neuroprotective properties, the neurotoxic effect of selenium has also been described (Vinceti et al., 2014).

Thus, disturbance of elemental status in children may contribute significantly to the etiology and pathogenesis of RAS. However, there is currently insufficient data indicating a causal relationship between micronutrient deficiencies and the development of RAS. Additional studies of elemental metabolism are needed to reveal the exact molecular mechanisms of its influence on the etiopathogenesis of RAS.

1.4 Neuroimmunologic shifts in RAS

S100B is a calcium-binding protein capable of forming dimers. It has numerous intra- and extracellular functions in norm and pathology. In the brain, S100B is produced mainly by astrocytes and, depending on the concentration, has trophic or toxic effects on neurons and glial cells.

S100 was discovered in 1965 as a fraction of brain glial proteins [85], which are produced mainly by astrocytes. Cerebral S100 is a combination of two closely related family proteins, S100A1 (S100α) and S100B (S100β) [23]. Since 1981 [18], S100 proteins have been identified in other tissues as well. By 2015, 20 members of the S100 family, intracellular calcium-sensing and calcium-binding proteins with a molecular weight of 10-12 kilodaltons, had been discovered [23, 72].

Among the 20 genes encoding S100 protein synthesis in humans, 16 are located in the q21 region of chromosome 1. These genes are designated as S100A (1, 2, ..., 16). The S100B gene is located in the q22 region of the 21st chromosome [72].

With some exceptions, S100 proteins exist inside the cell in the form of dimers. Thus, in the brain, S100A1 and S100B form homodimers S100A12 and S100B2, as well as heterodimers S100A1/S100B [51].

Due to their ability to regulate the activity of a number of proteins, S100A1 and S100B are involved in the transduction of signals controlling the activity of enzymes of energy metabolism in brain cells [60], calcium homeostasis [8], cell cycle, cytoskeleton functions [117], transcription [45], cell proliferation and differentiation [72], cell motility, secretory processes [72], and structural organization of biomembranes [23].

However, the most unusual characteristic of some members of the S100 family is their ability to be secreted extracellularly. S100-proteins in the extracellular sector exhibit properties of cytokines and interact with RAGE-receptors [6], which are expressed in the nervous system by neurons, microglia, astrocytes, and vascular wall cells [70].

Numerous findings of the last decade have allowed us to prove that glial cells not only provide structural support and trophicity of neurons, but also intensively interact with them. Due to the presence of ion channels as well as receptors to neurotransmitters and other signaling molecules in their distal outgrowths, astrocytes are able to register changes in neuronal activity [5] and respond by increasing the concentration of calcium in the cytosol [125] with the generation of calcium waves [79]. Further, the calcium signal is realized (probably, with the direct participation of S100) in modulation of expression of a number of genes, changes in the morphology of astrocytes and secretion by them of a number of neuroactive molecules, such as glutamate, D-serine, ATP, taurine, neurotrophins and cytokines [111, 120].

Astrocytes perform a wide range of adaptive functions, including neurotransmitter reuptake [22], aid in damage repair [109], and regulate synaptic density [132]. These findings suggest that glia-neuronal reciprocal signaling, functional and structural plasticity play a fundamental role in the operation of neuronal networks and information transfer/processing processes in the nervous system during its formation, function and repair.

One of the mediators in glia-neuronal and glia-glial interactions is S100B secreted by glial cells [2, 89].

As with most biologically active molecules, the effects of extracellular S100B are dose-dependent. In nanomolar concentrations, S100B has an autocrine effect on astrocytes, stimulating their proliferation in vitro [112], and the S100B2 dimer [56] modulates long-term synaptic plasticity [89], has a trophic effect on both developing [17, 56, 101, 122, 128] and regenerating neurons [9, 16].

In micromolar concentrations, extracellular S100B in the form of homo- and heterodimer can have neurotoxin effects on neurons and glia, inducing both apoptosis and cell necrosis [2, 47, 58]. The latter effect is based on the ability of S100B and independently induce proinflammatory cytokines, oxidative stress enzymes, in particular iNOS [47], and enhance other signals targeting neurons and glial cells [48].

S100B-induced enhancement of APP expression and iNOS activation may contribute to the generalization of inflammatory activation and neurodegeneration, as β-amyloid peptide can be secreted [7] and nitrogen monoxide (NO) can be diffused [47]. NO, in turn, can trigger the synthesis and release of other neurotoxic molecules from astrocytes, such as IL-8 and tumor necrosis factor alpha (TNF-α) [47].

Valuable data on the role of S100 in the functioning of the central nervous system (CNS) in norm and pathology have been obtained in experiments on animals in vivo. Thus, it was found that S100B plays a critical role in synaptogenesis, as its application to hippocampal neurons of mice induces the formation of synapses [88], and the introduction of antiserum to S100B into rat brain ventricles leads to a significant decrease in the density of synapses in the molecular layer of dentate gyrus [129].

The learning process (production of the food reflex) is accompanied by an increase in the content of S100 in the rat brain [40]. Injection of S100B into the rat hippocampus facilitates the formation of long-term memory [78], while administration of antiserum to S100 intracisternally or into the hippocampus inhibits LTP and leads to the loss of learned skills [40].

Proven correlations of S100B levels in biological fluids in various neurological and psychiatric disorders encourage to use its concentration as a surrogate biochemical indicator of primarily cognitive functioning in patients with lesions of the nervous system, as well as to monitor the effectiveness of therapy with its help [100].

Hippocampal axon/synaptic reorganization is another sign of MTLE, affecting "mossy" fibers of granular cells that contain neuropeptide Y, somostatin, and glutamate decarboxylase involved in GABA synthesis. MTLE patients with hippocampal sclerosis also have an increased level of mRNA factors NGF and BDGF in granular cells [49]. At the site of cortical damage after audiogenic seizures, astrocytes secrete an increased amount of GFAP. The number of GFAP-immunopositive astrocytes at the site of injury was increased by 25-37% compared to control and intact cortical area. The induction of GFAP suggests the participation of glia in compensatory NO-dependent mechanisms that are formed in the damaged cortical area during audiogenic attacks [136, 195].

When analyzing the results of histological and behavioral responses of mice to cerebral injury or kainate-induced seizures indicates a critical role for GFAP in hippocampal neurodegeneration after CNS lesions [104].

GFAP protein is the main structural component of intermediate filaments of astrocytes. It is known that changes in its expression are observed in various pathological processes involving brain glia (gliosis as a consequence of ischemic lesions, hemorrhage, trauma, toxic effects, etc.). [136].

The level of astroglial GFAP protein immunoreactivity and the number of GFAP-positive cells is a marker of neuronal loss in different molecular layers of the hippocampus down to the dentate gyrus, indicating a close relationship between neuronal and glial dysfunction [103, 153].

Thus, increased GFAP levels have been found to be a sensitive marker of brain damage.

Neurotrophic proteins also include nerve growth factor (NGF). Literature data on it are ambiguous. It is known that this protein is involved in maintaining the viability of central cholinergic neurons and sympathetic neurons of the peripheral (autonomous) nervous system. FRN is vital for the development of many neuronal populations in early ontogenesis [44, 217].

The following main groups of processes can be distinguished in neuroimmunopathology: immunoaggression, neurogenic immunodeficiency, and dysregulation of neuroimmune connections [34, 206]. The first, most intensively studied process should be considered the direct cytotoxic effect of autoantibodies and immunocytes sensitized to neuroantigens on the CNS. The second process - persistent neurogenic immunodeficiency - gives rise to neuroallergic processes. Close to the second process is the process of disruption of neuroimmune connections, caused by the action of various harmful factors on the corresponding regulatory links of the neuroimmune chain (metabolism of neurotransmitters and the state of receptors on neurons and immunocytes) [11, 51]. The latter process remains the least studied, despite the fact that it may be the cause of the continuous course and incurability of some neuroimmunopathologic processes. Mechanisms of immune system autoaggression against the CNS are involved in transplant rejection reactions or immediate and delayed type allergic reactions to various antigens [102, 133]. Three main criteria are used to prove the leading role of immunoaggression mechanisms in the pathogenesis of different forms of pathology: 1 Detection of immune complexes or lymphocyte-macrophage infiltrates in the foci of neural tissue damage, 2)cytotoxic effect on neural tissue in vitro by neurospecific antibodies or immunocytes sensitized to neuroantigens, 3) reproduction of an adequate model of the corresponding immunopathology in an experiment using antibodies or immune system cells [80, 158].

Immunologic mechanisms may be an important part of an integral theory of autism onset, and further immunologic studies will contribute to a better diagnosis of this disorder as well as open new therapeutic options.

1.5 Principles of microcurrent reflex therapy for autism in children

The treatment of ASD depends on factors that can level the very notion of "treatment". Differences in age, severity of impairment, comorbidities, family and community situation, availability of resources and economic development of society, provision of education (or lack thereof), medical and material assistance, opportunities for secure employment and non-discriminatory living upon reaching adulthood can be enormous [6,11,15].

Recent reviews of scientific publications indicate that few treatments meet the criteria for evaluating the effectiveness of interventions [8]. Nevertheless, the quality of evidence is improving, with a growing number of well-designed studies as well as randomized controlled trials [15]. However, even if the results are positive, most studies are still focused on short-term goals and limited outcome criteria. Few attempts are made to find answers to questions such as: is treatment effective in the long term or does it really improve patients' quality of life? Such problems may require very different research strategies, such as audits and reviews, systematic problem analysis and satisfaction assessments. It is also crucial to gather information about the attitudes and beliefs of people with ASD themselves.

Recently, microcurrent reflex therapy (MTRT) has been used in the treatment of children with RAS. MTRT is an effective modern method of treatment for a wide range of diseases, including CNS lesions in children, in particular for RAS.

According to a number of researchers, microstimulation leads to changes in the level of neuronal excitability, activation of conductive systems, provides adequate perception of exogenous and endogenous impulses by nerve cells, which is manifested by corresponding changes in the bioelectrical activity of the brain, parameters of somatosensory evoked potentials, reflex excitability of motoneurons, restoration of monosynaptic muscle reflex reactions to functional tests, improvement of motor, mental, speech and vegetative functions The listed mechanisms of microstimulation action on the CNS closely correlate with the currently revealed neuromorphological, neurophysiological and biochemical features of the pathogenesis of pediatric autism, which, presumably, can explain the effect of this therapeutic action [10]. MTRT occupies one of the leading places among non-medication methods of correction of cognitive and speech disorders in children.

RTT can improve the functioning of the parts of the brain responsible for speech and the desire for contact. However, there are few scientific studies evaluating the efficacy of RTT in children with ASD, and they are contradictory.

Conclusions of the chapter

The problem of studying autism spectrum disorders in childhood attracts increasing attention of researchers and general practitioners. Despite the rather multifaceted genetic, biochemical studies of diseases, in the structure of which atypical autism is most often found, it itself is essentially unsupported by the necessary descriptions of neurological status.

With the identified phenomenological "universality" of autism in childhood (Chigrinets A.N., 2015), as the commonality of its clinical manifestations in different diseases, it remains unclear what underlies this commonality, both from the neurological and pathogenetic positions. The methods of diagnostics of atypical autism and its therapy, taking into account the features of the underlying disease at different periods of its course, have not been sufficiently developed.

The etiology and pathogenesis of the disease are not currently understood. Autism spectrum disorders (ASD) are a set of neuropsychiatric disorders characterized by difficulties in social interactions and interest patterns, causing a wide range of disabilities. They typically manifest as speech impairments, repetitive and/or compulsive behaviors, hyperactivity, anxiety and difficulty adapting to new environments, and may also be accompanied by cognitive impairment [Anwar A et al., 2018; Rabbani N., Thornalley P.J., 2019]. The high heterogeneity of the clinical picture makes the diagnosis of RAS difficult and uncertain, especially in the early stages of the development of the disorder [Zwaigenbaum L., Penner M., 2018].

Recently, microcurrent reflex therapy (MTRT) has been used in the treatment of children with RAS. MTRT is an effective modern method of treatment for a wide range of diseases, including CNS lesions in children, particularly with RAS. It improves the functioning of the parts of the brain that are responsible for speech and the desire to communicate. However, there are few scientific studies evaluating the effectiveness of RTT in children with ASD and they are contradictory in nature.

CHAPTER II. GENERAL CHARACTERIZATION OF CLINICAL MATERIAL AND METHODS OF EXAMINATION

2.1 General characteristics of the observed children

The work was conducted at the Department of Neurology of the Tashkent Medical Institute and on the basis of the "ReoCenter" in the period from 2018 to 2021. The study included 405 children whose parents appealed with complaints about lack of sociability, speech, presence of stereotypical, repetitive behavior, limited interests and hobbies. The examination of the children was conducted in conjunction with a psychiatrist.

The study was conducted in 4 phases:

Stage 1 - 120 children with RAS were identified out of 405 children with complaints of lack of sociability, speech, stereotyped, repetitive behaviors, and limited interests and hobbies based on the M-CHAT-R screening interview method. The age of the children ranged from 2 to 6 years (mean age 3.8±0.4 years);

Stage 2 - according to M-CHAT-R data, clinical and neurological examination and on the basis of DSM- V criteria, 120 cases were diagnosed with RAS;

Stage 3 - hair micronutrients (61 children) and neuroprotein levels (80 children) in blood among children with RAS were analyzed;

Stage 4 - evaluation of the effectiveness of microcurrent reflexotherapy in the complex treatment of children with RAS. The children were divided into 2 groups by blind sampling method: the main group - 80 children included MTRT in the treatment complex, 40 children - standard pharmacotherapy and ABA-therapy. The effectiveness of therapy was assessed using the ATES and CARS questionnaires.

The diagnosis of ASD in the study groups was determined using the DSM-V criteria for diagnosing autistic disorder (Table 2.1). For domain A, all 3 symptoms must be present, and for domain B, 2 of the 4 symptoms must be present.

Table 2.1.

DSM-5 diagnostic criteria for autism spectrum disorder

Domains	Criteria: deficits
A. Persistent impairment in social communication and social interaction in different contexts, presently or in the past in the following ways; all 3 symptoms from this domain must be present	1. Reciprocal social interaction.
	2. Nonverbal communicative behaviors used for social interaction.
	3. Ability to establish and maintain relationships and understand their essence.
	Establishment of 1 criterion
	Combination of 2 criteria
	Combination of 3 criteria
B. Limited, repetitive patterns of behavior, interests, or actions manifested currently or in the past in at least 2 of the following forms;	1. Stereotyped or repetitive movements, use of objects or speech.
	2. The patient insists on constancy, is inflexible about new things, is strict about adherence to established routines, and uses ritualized patterns of verbal and nonverbal behavior.
	3. Extremely limited, fixed interests manifested with atypical intensity and focus.
	4. Hyper- or hypo-sensitivity to sensory stimuli or unusual interests in sensory aspects of the environment.
	Establishment of 1 criterion
	Combination of 2 criteria
	Combination of 3 criteria
	Combination of 4 criteria

The following groups were formed to fulfill the goal and solve the tasks. The control group consisted of 30 children, comparable to the main group by sex and age, attending educational institutions and having no autistic disorders (Fig. 2.1). The main group consisted of 120 children with ASD.

Exclusion criteria from the above groups were: current organic lesions of the central nervous system (CNS); hereditary metabolic disorders (phenylketonuria, tyrosinemia, hyperglycyuria, etc.); chromosomal diseases; other (other) autism spectrum disorders.

2.2 Research Methods

Characterization of nosological groups of patients is supplemented by information about the pathology of pregnancy and childbirth in the mothers of patients, as well as the presence of pathology of the neonatal period.

Neurological examination was performed, consistently assessing the state of higher brain functions, cranial nerves (CNN), motor function (voluntary movements, coordination, involuntary movements), sensitivity, meningeal syndrome, and autonomic-trophic functions.

Many questionnaires have been developed that can be used as tools for assessing children's development, as well as for screening RAS, and various algorithms for its implementation have been proposed. However, the M-CHAT-R screening method, supplemented by the M-CHAT interview, is the most optimal. M-CHAT -Modified CHecklist for Autismin Toddlers, a modified questionnaire for autism in young children (Robins, Fein, Barton&Green, 2011).

This is actually a pre-screening, after which groups with a significantly higher risk of developing RAS and with identified symptoms of RAS are formed. Wetherby et al. (2015), for example, use a minimum number of well-defined features in the pre-screening phase:

1. absence of humming until 12 months of age;

2. absence of gesticulation up to 12 months of age;

3. The child does not utter a single word before 16 months of age;

4. lack of meaningful (not echolalic) two-word phrases by 24 months of age;

5. Any impairment of speech or social skills at any age.

A 20-item questionnaire for parents or caregivers; ages 16-30 mo, takes up to 20 min.

Scoring Algorithm. For all items except 2, 5, and 12, a "NO" response indicates RAS risk; for items 2, 5, and 12, a "YES" response indicates RAS risk. The following algorithm maximizes the psychometric properties of the M-CHAT-R:

Low risk: Total score is 0-2; if the child is younger than 24 months, check again after the second birthday. If there is no risk of RAS, no further action is required.

Medium Risk: Total score is 3-7; follow-up questions (Stage 2 M-CHAT-R/F) are administered to obtain additional information about the level of risk. The following actions are required: conduct a diagnostic assessment of the child and the appropriateness of early intervention.

If the follow-up count shows 0-1, the result of the examination is considered negative. No further action is required if a risk of RAS is identified, but the child should be re-screened at follow-up visits.

High Risk: Total score is 8-20; it is acceptable to skip follow-up questions and move immediately to diagnostic evaluation and appropriateness of early intervention.

№	Questions	Yes	No
1	If you point to an object in the room, does your child look at it? (For *example,* if you point to a toy or an animal, does your child look at the toy or animal?)		

2	Has it ever occurred to you that your child is deaf?		
3	Does your child like to pretend? (*For example, pretending* to drink from an empty cup, talking on the phone, feeding a doll or toy animal?)		
4	Does your child like to climb objects? (*For example,* furniture, playground, stairs?)		
5	Does your child make unusual finger movements near the head and eyes? (*For example, does he/she* wiggle his/her fingers near the eyes?)		
6	Does your child point his/her finger when he/she wants to ask for something or asks for help? (*For example, does he/she point to a* snack or toy he/she can't reach?)		
7	Does your child use one finger to point to something interesting that he/she wants to point out to you? (*For example, an* airplane in the sky or a big truck on the road?)		
8	Is your child interested in other children? (*For example,* does your child look at, laugh at, or approach other children?)		
9	Does your child bring you things to look at, show you things - not to help you, but just to share? (*For example, does your child show you a* flower, a toy animal, a toy truck?)		
10	Does your child respond when you call his/her name? (*For example,* does he/she look at you, talk or babble, stop what he/she is doing when he/she hears his/her name?)		
11	When you smile at your child, does he or she smile back?		
12	Does your child get upset by household noises? (For example, does he/she scream or cry in response to the noise of a vacuum cleaner or loud music?)		
13	Is your child walking?		

1 4	Does your child look you in the eye when you talk to him/her, play with him/her, or dress him/her?		
1 5	Does your child try to copy what you do? (*For example,* waving, clapping hands, making funny noises after you)		
1 6	If you turn your head to look at something, does your child look around to see what you are looking at?		
1 7	Does your child try to get you to look at him/her? (*For example, does your child look at you* to hear praise, say "look" or "look at me"?)		
1 8	Does your child understand when you tell him/her to do something? (*For example,* if you don't point to an object, can your child understand the words "put the book on the chair" or "bring me a blanket"?)		
1 9	If something new is happening, does your child look you in the face to see exactly how you feel about it (*For example,* if he hears a strange or funny noise, or sees a new toy, will he look you in the face?).		
2 0	Does your child like moving activities? (*For example,* being tossed or rocked on your knee)		
	Bottom line:		

To assess the dynamics of children's condition during observation and treatment in this study, the CARS scale [Schopler E. et al., 1980, 1988; translated by Elina &Uri], which is a widely used assessment scale in the United States to determine the severity of autistic manifestations in children from 3 to 15 years of age, was used.

The scale includes 15 items characterizing all areas of child functioning that are important for the survey. These include "desire for contact with others", "ability to imitate", "features of emotional reactions", "motor skills", "use of play and nonplay objects", "adaptation to change", "visual reactions", "auditory reactions", "gustatory, olfactory and tactile reactions", "presence of fears and anxiety", "speech features", "nonverbal interaction", "nonverbal interaction", and "visual, auditory and tactile reactions", olfactory and tactile reactions", "presence of fears and anxiety", "speech features", "non-verbal interaction", "degree and productivity of activity", "level and features of intellectual development", "evaluation of the clinician's overall impression".

In the process of testing, each of these parameters is compared with the corresponding indicators of the age norm, and all features of the child's behavior that fall outside the normal age limits are assessed. Testing on this scale can be carried out taking into account any information available at the moment (along with the direct assessment of the child's behavior at the reception, the results of experimental-psychological research, as well as information received from parents and teachers can be taken into account).

According to this scale, the severity of autism was determined in points. The final score in the range from 15 to 29 points corresponds to the absence of autism, mild/moderately pronounced autism - 30-36 points, severe autism - 37-60 points.

To assess the effectiveness of therapy for children with RAS, the ATEC test was administered. The ATEC is a one-page form designed to be completed by parents or physicians. The test consists of 4 subtests: I. Speech / language communication (14 items); II. Communication skills (20 items); III. Sensory / cognitive awareness (18 items); and IV. Health / physical condition / behavior (25 items).

The ATES score in the dynamics of observation was evaluated as follows: if a child with RAS initially scored 40 points, and after a month 35 points, then in this case there is an improvement, but if the scores increase from the initial scores - then deterioration.

Iterpretation of ATES test scores:

10 – 15	не аутичный ребенок, полностью нормальный, хорошо развитый ребенок
16 – 30	не аутичный ребенок, небольшие отклонения в сторону задержки развития
31 – 40	мягкая или умеренная степень аутизма
41 – 60	средняя степень аутизма
61 и выше	тяжелый аутизм

2.3 Hair microelement composition

Hair for analysis was cut with scissors from 3-5 sites on the occipital part of the head according to IAEA recommendations. The length of hair from the root to the distal part was 2-4 cm. The cut hairs were washed thoroughly in acetone, dried, weighed and packed in labeled polyethylene bags. The prepared samples were subjected to neutron activation analysis.

Methodology of neutron-activation determination of elements in hair. Instrumental neutron activation analysis allows to determine more than 20 elements in one sample. At the same time for their determination it is necessary to resort to multiple irradiation and rather long measurement time. To determine the content of elements for nuclides with different half-lives, it is necessary to apply different time modes of analysis (irradiation, cooling, and measurement times). The different modes require either separate sample suspensions or the use of a single sample suspension for repeated irradiations, which increases the analysis time due to the need to wait for the decay of short-lived nuclides after the first irradiation. After studying the characteristic gamma spectra of activated samples, we proposed the following modes:

1. irradiation time 15 sec, cooling time 5 min, measurement time 100 sec,

2. irradiation time 15 sec, cooling time 2 hours, measurement time 100 sec

3. irradiation time 15 h, cooling time 7 days, measurement time 200 sec

4. irradiation time 15 h, cooling time 20 days, measurement time 400 sec.

The developed techniques for neutron-activation determination of elements are as follows:

Determination of sodium, chlorine, manganese, copper and iodine: Samples together with standards were packed in a polyethylene container and irradiated in the vertical channel of the reactor with a neutron flux of 5.10^{13} neutron/cm^2 .sec for 15 sec. The induced activity was measured twice - through the

Table 2.2.

Nuclear-physical characteristics of the determined elements and parameters of the developed methods.

Element	Nuclide	Gamma-quantum energy,kev	Half-life	Determination limit, µg/g
Na	24-Na	1369	15 hr.	5
Cl	38-Cl	1642	37.2 min.	100
Ca	47-Sc.	160	3.43 days.	250
Sc	46-Sc.	889	84 days	0,001
Cr	51-Cr.	320	27.2 days.	0,08
Mn	56-Mn	845	2.58 hours.	0,05
Fe	59-Fe.	1098	44.5 days.	10
Co	60-Co.	1173	5.27 years.	0,01
Cu	64-Cu	511	12.8 hours.	1.0
Zn	65-Zn	1115	244 days	5.0
Se	75-Se.	265	120 days	0,05
Br	82-Br.	777	1.47 hours.	0,1
Ag	110m-Ag	658	250 days.	0,01
Sb	124-Sb.	1696	60 days	0,01
I	128-I	443	25.4 min.	0,1
La	140-La.	1595	40.2 hours.	0,01
Au	198-Au.	411	2.69 days.	0,001
Hg	203-Hg.	278	46.6 days.	0,01
U	230-Np.	228	2.35 days.	0,02

5-10 min after irradiation for the determination of iodine and chlorine and 2 hours later for the determination of sodium, copper and manganese.

Determination of calcium, bromine, lanthanum, gold and uranium: For determination of calcium, bromine, lanthanum, gold and uranium content the same samples were wrapped in aluminum foil and irradiated in the wet channel of the reactor for 15 hours. The induced activity was measured 7 days after irradiation for the corresponding nuclides given in Table 2.3.

Table 2.3.

Evaluation of the correctness of the analysis results

Element	Certified content, µg/g	Found by us, µg/g	Relative deviation,%
Ag	0.19± 0.06	0.21± 0.064	+10
Au	0.03± 0.01	0.026± 0.007	-12
Br	4.16± 2.1	4.3± 0.54	+2.4
Ca	522± 160	540± 120	+3.6
Cl	2265± 71	2280± 71	+0.7
Co	5.97± 1.2	5.48± 0.49	-8.1
Cr	0.27± 0.16	0.28± 0.08	+3.8
Cu	10± 3.2	13± 2.9	+30
Hg	1.7± 0.24	1.8± 0.5	+6
Fe	24± 9.8	26± 4.8	+9
I	2.0± 0.89	2.3± 0.37	+12
La	0.01± 0.01	0.012± 0.007	+20
Mn	0.85± 0.25	0.8± 0.07	-5.9
Sb	0.03± 0.01	0.033± 0.01	+10
Se	0.35± 0.04	0.32± 0.062	+8.4
U	0.14± 0.015	0.16± 0.03	+13
Zn	174± 32	180± 15	+3.4

Determination of scandium, chromium, iron, cobalt, zinc, selenium, silver, rubidium, antimony and mercury: To determine the content of the above elements, samples irradiated for 15 h were measured one month after irradiation for the respective radionuclides.

All measurements were performed on a germanium detector and spectrometer path connected to a PC.

Various standards were used to determine the elemental content: in-laboratory standards obtained by applying a known amount of the element on an anhydrous filter paper and IAEA standard comparison samples H-4 (Animalblood) and HH-1 (hair homogenate), as well as the comparator method.

2.4 Neuroimmunologic studies

Quantitative determination of serum immunoreactivity of neurotropic autoantibodies of IgG class (natural neurotropic autoantibodies - AT1 and their functional counterbalances - anti-idiotypic antibodies - AIAT2) directed to nervous tissue proteins NF200, GFAP, S100, OBM, B-channel, Hol-R, Glu-R, DA-R, Ser-R, DNA, B2 GP) was performed in blood serum samples of all observed patients, as well as in blood samples of clinically healthy individuals (control group - n=16).Ca-channel, Hol-R, Glu-R, GABA-R, DA-R, Ser-R, DNA, B2 GP.

Determination of the content of neurotropic autoantibodies (NAAT) was performed using standard procedures of solid-phase immunoassay ELI-N-Test and test kits of the same name produced by MIC "Immunculus" (Russia) according to the method of A.B. Poletaev (1988; 1995; 2017). The method allows to detect abnormalities in the serum content of autoantibodies of IgG class of certain antigenic specificity. The reactions of the "internal standard" with each antigen were performed on each of the plates (Poletaev A.B., Russian Federation Patent #2147128, 2000).

To quantify changes in the relative content of autoantibodies to NF200, GFAP, S100, OBM, their individual content in 30 duplicate samples of analyzed sera was calculated in order to calculate individual deviations of autoantibody immunoreactivity of a certain specificity from the individual mean immunoreactivity level of each patient (expressed as %% of the total mean). To do this:

1. The arithmetic mean values of OD values in reaction with each antigen were calculated for the control serum and for the analyzed serum samples.

2. The average individual immunoreactivity of each analyzed serum sample with all antigens used was calculated using the formula:

$$СИР = \left(\frac{R(ar1) \times 100}{R(k1)} - 100 + \frac{R(ar2) \times 100}{R(k2)} - 100 + \ldots\ldots + \frac{R(ar12) \times 100}{R(k12)} - 100 \right) : 12$$

Where:

SIR - average individual serum immunoreactivity of a particular patient, expressed as a percentage of population average (control) values;

R(ar1, 2, ...12) - value of optical density of analyzed blood serum in wells with antigens-1, 2, ...12;

R(k1, 2, ...12) - value of optical density of control serum in wells with antigens-1, 2, ...12.

3. The deviations (in percent of the mean normalized level) of immunoreactivity of the analyzed blood serum sample with each of the antigens used were calculated according to the formula:

$$R(норм)\ ar1 = \left(\frac{ОП(ar1) \times 100}{ОП(k1)} \right) - 100 - СИР$$

$$R(норм)\ ar2 = \left(\frac{ОП(ar2) \times 100}{ОП(k2)} \right) - 100 - СИР$$

$$R(норм)\ ar12 = \left(\frac{ОП(ar12) \times 100}{ОП(k12)} \right) - 100 - СИР$$

Where:

R (norms) ar1, ar2, ... ar12 - deviations (in percent of the average normalized level) of immunoreactivity of the analyzed blood serum sample with antigen-1, antigen-2, ... antigen-12;

OD (ar1, 2, ...12) - optical density of reaction of blood serum sample with antigens ar1, ar2, ... ar12;

OP (k1, 2, ... 12) is the optical density of the reaction of control serum with antigens ar1, ar2, ... ar12;

SIR - average individual serum immunoreactivity of a particular patient, expressed as a percentage of population average (control) values.

4. When taking into account the results, the authors of the ELI-Test technique proposed the optimum of the values of the average individual level of immunoreactivity (in comparison with the control), which is in the range of -20% ... +10% of the average level of reaction of control serum with the antigens used. It was calculated according to the formula p.2.

The level of serum AAT to each antigen was expressed in conditional units (CU): percent of deviations from the standard serum IR. AAT immunoreactivity values from 80 to 140 U.U. and AT1/AIAT2 immunoreactivity index from 0.8 to 1.2 were considered normal [9,16].

2.5 Statistical methods of research

The obtained data were subjected to statistical processing on a Pentium-4 personal computer using programs developed in EXCEL package, using a library of statistical functions, with calculation of arithmetic mean (M), standard deviation (σ), standard error (m), relative values (frequency, %), Student's criterion (t), with calculation of probability of error (P). Correlation analysis was performed according to the method of K. Spearman and M. Kendel.

Statistical analysis of the results was performed using the statistical software package "OpenEpi 2009, Version 2.3" and *"Doctor Stat 2013,*

Version 1.9". In case of differences between the control and the study group, the odds ratio (OR) with 95% CI confidence interval was calculated.

Differences in mean values were considered reliable at a significance level of $P<0.05$. The existing guidelines for statistical processing of clinical and laboratory tests results were followed (Zaitsev V.M. et al., 2014).

CHAPTER 3. EARLY DIAGNOSIS AND CLINICAL AND NEUROLOGICAL CHARACTERISTICS OF AUTISM SPECTRUM DISORDERS IN CHILDREN

3.1 Early diagnosis of autism spectrum disorders using the MCHAT-R screening questionnaire

Stage 1 of the study was to identify children with RAS. As a result, we conducted the M-CHAT-R screening diagnostic method among 405 children with suspected RAS.

Children came in complaining of lack of sociability, speech, having stereotypical, repetitive behaviors, and limited interests and hobbies.

The percentages of Yes and No scores on the M-CHAT-R screening test are given in Table 3.1.

Table 3.3.

Results of the M-CHAT-R screening diagnostic method in children with suspected RAS

№	Questions	Yes		No	
		n	%	n	%
1	If you point to an object in the room, does your child look at it? (For *example,* if you point to a toy or an animal, does your child look at the toy or animal?)	263	65,0	142	35,0
2	Has it ever occurred to you that your child is deaf?	20	5,0	385	95,0
3	Does your child like to pretend? (*For example, pretending* to drink from an empty cup, talking on the phone, feeding a doll or toy animal?)	243	60,0	162	40,0
4	Does your child like to climb objects? (*For example,* furniture, playground, stairs?)	385	95,0	20	5,0
5	Does your child make unusual finger movements near the head and eyes? (*For example, does he/she* wiggle his/her fingers near the eyes?)	223	55,0	182	45,0
6	Does your child point his/her finger when he/she wants to ask for something or asks for help? (*For example, does he/she point to a* snack or toy he/she can't reach?)	243	60,0	162	40,0
7	Does your child use one finger to point to something interesting that he/she wants to point	243	60,0	162	40,0

	out to you? (*For example, an* airplane in the sky or a big truck on the road?)				
8	Is your child interested in other children? (*For example,* does your child look at, laugh at, or approach other children?)	142	35,0	263	65,0
9	Does your child bring you things to look at, show you things - not to help you, but just to share? (*For example, does your child show you a* flower, a toy animal, a toy truck?)	203	50,0	203	50,0
10	Does your child respond when you call his/her name? (*For example,* does he/she look at you, talk or babble, stop what he/she is doing when he/she hears his/her name?)	344	85,0	61	15,0
11	When you smile at your child, does he or she smile back?	405	100,0	0	0,0
12	Does your child get upset by household noises? (For example, does he/she scream or cry in response to the noise of a vacuum cleaner or loud music?)	182	45,0	223	55,0
13	Is your child walking?	405	100,0	0	0,0
14	Does your child look you in the eye when you talk to him/her, play with him/her, or dress him/her?	304	75,0	101	25,0
15	Does your child try to copy what you do? (*For example,* waving, clapping hands, making funny noises after you)	324	80,0	81	20,0
16	If you turn your head to look at something, does your child look around to see what you are looking at?	142	35,0	263	65,0
17	Does your child try to get you to look at him/her? (*For example, does your child look at you* to hear praise, say "look" or "look at me"?)	344	85,0	61	15,0
18	Does your child understand when you tell him/her to do something? (*For example,* if you don't point to an object, can your child understand the words "put the book on the chair" or "bring me a blanket"?)	223	55,0	182	45,0
19	If something new is happening, does your child look you in the face to see exactly how you feel about it (*For example,* if he hears a strange or funny noise, or sees a new toy, will he look you in the face?).	162	40,0	243	60,0
20	Does your child like moving activities? (*For example,* being tossed or rocked on your knee)	405	100,0	0	0

The results of the study showed that 44.9% of children (n=182) were found to be at low risk. Parents of children with low risk level of ASD answered "No" to such questions as "Have you ever thought that your child might be deaf?", "Does your child make unusual finger movements near the head and eyes?", "Does your child get upset by unusual finger movements near the head and eyes? , "Does your child make unusual finger movements near the head and eyes?", "Does your child get upset by household noises?". At the same time, they answered "Yes" to such questions as "If you point to an object in the room, does your child look at it?", "Does your child play imaginary or role-playing games?", "Does your child like to climb on objects?", "Does your child point to something interesting to draw your attention to it?", "Is your child interested in other children?", "Does your child show you objects by bringing them to you or holding them near you, just to share rather than asking for help?", "Does your child respond when you call his/her name?", "When you smile at your child, does he/she smile back at you?", "Can your child walk?", "Does your child look you in the eye when you talk, play or dress him/her?", "Does your child try to copy what you do?", "If you turn your head to look at something, does your child look around to see what you are looking at?", "If you turn your head to look at something, does your child look around to see what you are looking at?", "Does your child try to make you look at him/her?", "Does your child understand when you tell him/her to do something?", "If something new is happening, does your child look at your face to see how you feel about it?", "Does your child like moving activities?".

The average risk level was revealed in 30.1% of children (n=122). Parents of children at average risk for ASD answered "Yes" to questions such as "Does your child like to climb on objects?", "Does your child point to something interesting to get your attention?", "Does your child point to ask for something or get help?", "Does your child respond when you call his/her name?", "When you smile at your child, does he/she smile back at you?", "Does your child know how to walk?", "Does your child try to copy what you do?", "If you turn your head to look at something, does your child look around to see what you are looking at?", "Does your child try to make you look at him/her?", "Does your child understand when you tell him/her to do something?", "If something new happens, does your child look at your face to see how you feel about it?", "Does your child like moving activities?". At the same time they answered "No" to such questions as "If you point to an object in the room, does your child look at it?", "Have you ever thought that your child might be deaf?", "Does your child play imaginary or role-playing games?", "Does your child make unusual movements with fingers near the head and eyes?", "Is your child interested in other children?", "Does your child show you objects by bringing them to you or holding them near you just to share rather than asking for help?", "Does your child get upset by household noises?", "Does your child look you in the eye when you talk to him/her, play with him/her, or dress him/her?".

The analysis revealed a high risk level in 24.9% of surveyed children (n=101), whose parents answered "Yes" to such questions as "Does your child play imaginary or role-playing games?", "Does your child like to climb on objects?", "Does your child make unusual finger movements near the head and eyes?", "Does your child respond when you call his/her name?", "When you smile at your child, does he/she smile back?", "Does your child get upset by household noises?", "Does your child know how to walk?", "Does your child look you in the eye when you talk, play or dress him/her?", "Does your child try to copy what you do?", "Does your child try to make you look at him/her?", "Does your child like moving activities?".At the same time, they answered "No" to such questions as "If you point to an object in the room, does your child look at it?", "Have you ever thought that your child might be deaf?", "Does your child point to ask for something or get help?", "Does your child point to something interesting to get your attention?", "Is your child interested in other children?", "Does your child show you objects by bringing them to you or holding them near you, just to share, not to ask for help?", "If you turn the holo

Thus, the prevalence of medium and high risk of developing RAS according to the screening questionnaire M-CHAT-R (30.1% and 24.9%, respectively) was found among the 405 children examined.

As a result of further examination, according to DSM-5 criteria, we found that at low risk of RAS according to the M-CHAT-R questionnaire, RAS was not diagnosed in 100% of cases, at medium risk - RAS was diagnosed in 15.6% of children, while at high risk of RAS - RAS was diagnosed in 100% of cases (Table 3.2).

Table 3.2.

DSM-5 diagnostic criteria for autism spectrum disorder

Domains	Criteria: deficits	Number of patients					
		Low risk of RAS (n=182)		Average RAS risk (n=122)		High risk of RAS (n=101)	
		n	%	n	%	n	%
A. Persistent impairment in social communication and social interaction in different contexts, presently or in the past in the following ways; all 3 symptoms from this domain must be present	1. Reciprocal social-social interaction.	25	13,7	57	46,7	10 1	100,0
	2. Nonverbal communicative behaviors used for social interaction.	56	30,8	28	23,0	10 1	100,0
	3. Ability to establish and maintain relationships, understand their essence.	10 1	55,5	56	45,9	10 1	100,0
	Establishment of 1 criterion	15 8	86,8	85	69,7	0	0,0
	Combination of 2 criteria	24	13,2	18	14,8	0	0,0
	Combination of 3 criteria	**0**	**0,0**	**19**	**15,6**	**10 1**	**100,0**
B. Restricted, repetitive patterns of behavior, interests, or actions presently or in the past in at least 2 of the following forms; 2 of the 4 symptoms must be present.	1. Stereotyped or repetitive movements, use of objects or speech.	67	36,8	52	42,6	52	51,5
	2. The patient insists on constancy, is inflexible with respect to new things, strictly follows the established routine, uses ritualized	58	31,9	49	40,2	47	46,5

	patterns of verbal and non-verbal behavior.					
	3. Extremely limited, fixed interests, manifested with atypical intensity and focus.	0	0,0	19	15,6	39	38,6
	4. Hyper- or hypo-sensitivity to sensory stimuli or unusual interests in sensory aspects of the environment.	57	31,3	21	17,2	18	17,8
	Establishment of 1 criterion	182	100,0	103	84,4	0	0,0
	Combination of 2 criteria	**0**	**0,0**	**14**	**11,5**	**74**	**73,3**
	Combination of 3 criteria	**0**	**0,0**	**5**	**4,1**	**12**	**11,9**
	Combination of 4 criteria	**0**	**0,0**	**0**	**0,0**	**15**	**14,9**

Thus, out of 405 children examined, 120 children were diagnosed with RAS, which amounted to 29.6%. The sensitivity of the M-CHAT-R screening method is 95.1%, specificity 90.3%, and accuracy 91.3% (Fig. 3.1).

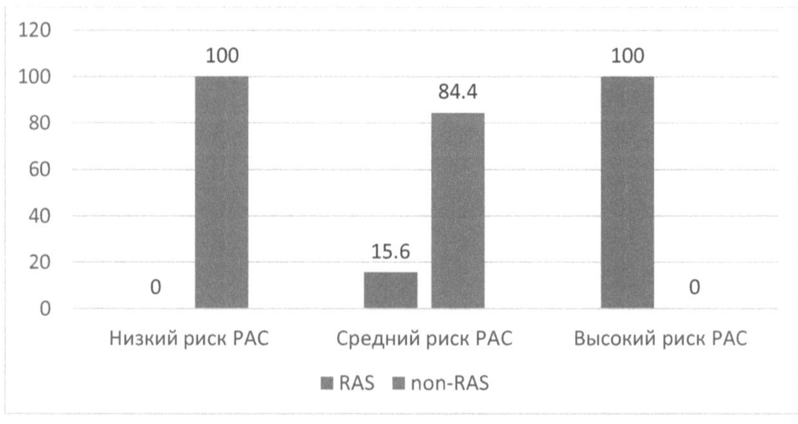

Figure 3.1. Evaluation of sensitivity and specificity of the M-CHAT-R screening questionnaire using DSM-5 criteria

In connection with the above data, we recommend this method as a screening for early diagnosis of RAS in children aged 2 to 6 years.

Based on the above, we have developed criteria for early diagnosis of RAS using the results of M Chat and DSM 5 (Khusenova N.T., Majidova E.N., Ergasheva N.N., 2023)

3.2 Clinical and neurological features of children with RAS

Based on the above, 120 children with RAS were examined.

The next stage of our work is to assess the clinical, anamnestic and neurological status of 120 children with RAS. Thus, we found that the peak of RAS detection falls at the age of 4-6 years. According to the distribution by sex, we found an almost 4-fold predominance of boys over girls in all age groups (Fig. 3.2).

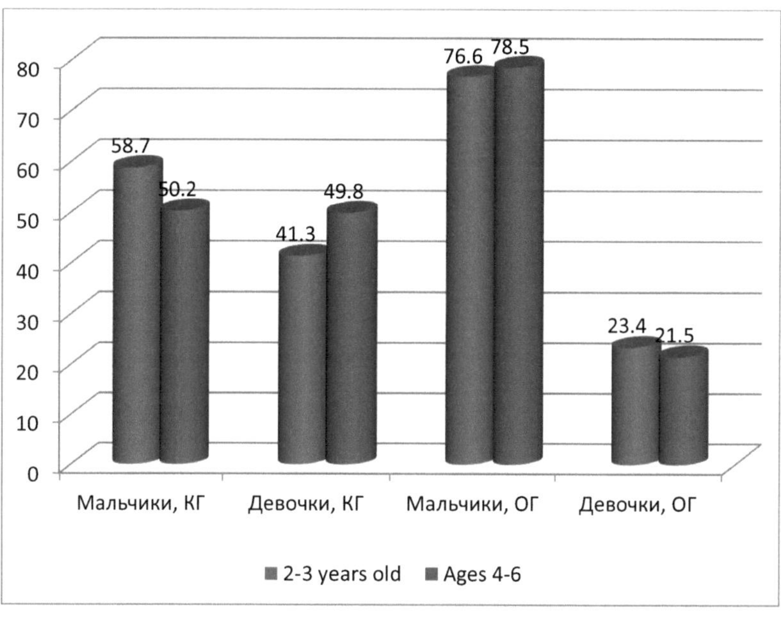

Figure 3.2. **Age gradation of the examined RAS children (n=120)**

Дети с жалобами на отсутствие коммуникабельности, речи, наличие стереотипных, повторяющееся поведение, ограниченные интересы и увлечения		
Скрининговый метода опроса M-CHAT-R		
Для всех пунктов, кроме 2, 5 и 12, ответ «НЕТ» указывает на риск РАС; для пунктов 2, 5 и 12 на риск РАС указывает ответ «ДА».		
Низкий риск	**Средний риск**	**Высокий риск**
Общий счет составляет 0-2; если ребенок младше 24 месяцев, проверьте его снова после второго года рождения. В случае отсутствия риска РАС дальнейших действий не требуется.	Общий счет составляет 3-7; назначаются последующие вопросы (второй этап M-CHAT-R/F) для получения дополнительной информации о степени риска. Требуются следующие действия: провести диагностическое оценивание ребенка и приемлемости раннего вмешательства. Если последующий подсчет показывает 0-1, результат осмотра считается отрицательным. Не требуется дальнейших действий, если выявлен риск РАС, но во время последующих визитов ребенок должен быть проверен повторно.	Общий счет составляет 8-20; допустимо пропустить последующие вопросы и незамедлительно перейти к диагностической оценке и целесообразности раннего вмешательства.
Дальнейшая диагностика и лечение основного заболевания	**Проведение оценки по критериям DSM- V**	
	А. Устойчивые нарушения в социальной коммуникации и социальном взаимодействии в различных контекстах, проявляемые в настоящий момент или в прошлом в указанных далее формах. 1. Реципрокное социальное взаимодействие 2. Невербальное коммуникативное поведение, используемое для социального взаимодействия. 3. Способность завязывать и поддерживать взаимоотношения, понимать их сущность.	В. Ограниченные, повторяющиеся шаблоны поведения, интересы или действия, проявляемые в настоящий момент или в прошлом как минимум в 2-х из указанных далее форм: 1. Стереотипные или повторяющиеся движения, использование объектов или речи; 2. Пациент настаивает на постоянстве, негибок в отношении нового, строго следит за соблюдением установленного распорядка, использует ритуализованные шаблоны вербального и невербального поведения; 3. Крайне ограниченные, фиксированные интересы, проявляющиеся с нетипичной интенсивностью и сосредоточенностью. 4. Гипер- или гипо-чувствительность к сенсорным стимулам либо необычные интересы к сенсорным аспектам среды.
Домен А - должны быть в наличии все 3 симптома из этого домена		
Домен В - должны быть в наличии 2 из 4-х симптомов.		
Нет в наличии		Есть в наличии
Дальнейшая диагностика и лечение основного заболевания		**Диагноз РАС**

Criteria for early diagnosis of RAS using M Chat and DSM 5 results (Khusenova N.T., Majidova E.N., Ergasheva N.N., 2023)

The study of hereditary predisposition (Table 3.3) revealed an aggravated history of mental illness among children with ASD (p < 0.05). These data are of particular interest, as they once again prove that there are genetic predisposition factors in the development of autism.

Table 3.3.

Frequency of psychiatric and degenerative CNS diseases in relatives of children from the studied groups, abs. (%)

groups	Not burdened	Aggravation for mental illnesses	Aggravation for degenerative diseases
control, n = 35	85,7	8,6	5,7
RAS, n = 120	68,9	27,1	4,1

Note: * - statistically significant differences at p < 0.05

The neurological status at the time of examination of the children was characterized by diffuse microsymptomatology in the form of tonus dissociation, changes in reflexes (mild asymmetry of tendon and periosteal reflexes), low speech production and the presence of a defect in social communication (Fig. 3.3).

Cranial nerves - insufficiency of cranial innervation in the form of asymmetry and smoothness of nasolabial folds, asymmetry of eye slits, deviation of the tongue from the midline, etc.; convergence and accommodation disorders were present in 15.6% of children; smoothness and less mobility of the nasolabial fold: right - 17.2% of children, left - 12.4% of children.Convergence and accommodation disorders were found in 15.6% of children, smoothing and less mobility of the nasolabial fold: right - in 17.2% of children, left - in 12.4% of children; tongue deviation from the midline in 35% (most children refused to follow this instruction), bulbar and pseudobulbar symptoms were not detected, but 37.5% of children showed prolonged retention of food in the mouth with a preserved swallowing reflex.

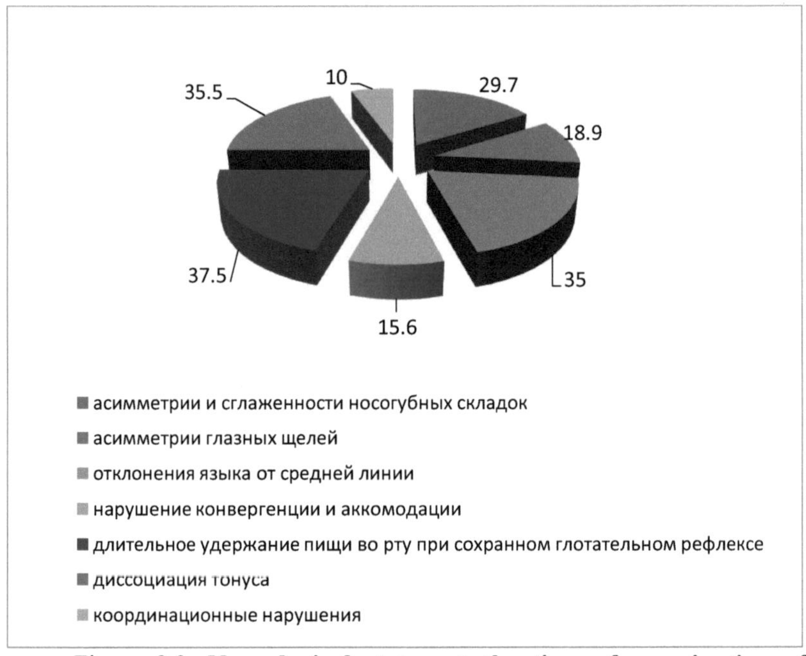

Figure 3.3. **Neurological status at the time of examination of children with RAS**

Dissociation of tone, pathologic reflexes, and coordination disorders were in 35.5-10.0%.

In the structure of neurologic pathology (Table 3.4), we considered individual neurologic syndromes such as peripheral cervical insufficiency, muscular dystonia syndrome, pyramidal-extrapyramidal insufficiency syndrome, enuresis, and other syndromes (tics, seizure syndrome, hypertension-hydrocephalic syndrome).

Table 3.4.

Structure of neurological syndromes (in % of the total number of children with these diseases), abs. (%)

Nosologic forms	Control group (n = 35)		Main group (n = 120)	
Peripheral cervical insufficiency syndrome.	5	14,2	19	19
Muscular dystonia syndrome	7	20	25	25
Pyramidal, extrapyramidal symptoms.	2	5,7	16	16
Enuresis	1	2,8	8	8
Sleep disorders	2	5,7	41	41
Other syndromes	5	14,2	6	6
No CNS pathology	15	42,8	9	9

Note: * - differences are statistically significant at p < 0.05.

It was revealed that children with RAS have a significantly (p<0.05) higher frequency of sleep disorders (dyssomnias, insomnias, somnolongia, somnambulism, nightmares) - 41%.

It is also noted that the percentage of children with no pathologic changes in the CNS is statistically significantly (p<0.05) lower compared to controls (42.8%, vs. 9%).

Based on the above, we can assume that, according to our results, these syndromes (pyramidal and extrapyramidal insufficiency syndrome, muscular dystonia syndrome, enuresis and others) may be a consequence of a fairly high frequency of subclinical forms of central nervous system damage in the perinatal period.

Neuropsychological examination complemented the neurological examination, significantly increasing the efficiency of topical diagnosis of brain lesions and interhemispheric interaction. In order to clarify the mechanism of symptom formation, as well as to analyze the state and dynamics of development of mental functions in different variants of speech development disorder, we conducted a neuropsychological study. The revealed neuropsychological disorders of higher brain functions in the examined children are presented in Fig. 3.4.

The neuropsychological study included assessment of kinesthetic, dynamic and spatial praxis, auditory-motor coordination, stereognosis, visual gnosis, speech, auditory-speech memory, drawing and visual memory.

Speech disorders were found in 100% of cases in both groups. In the main group, auditory gnosis, astereognosis, auditory-motor coordination and dynamic praxis were significantly predominant (87%, 83%, 83% and 77%, respectively). At the same time, these disorders were significantly less in the comparison group (57%, 43%, 30% and 23%, respectively).

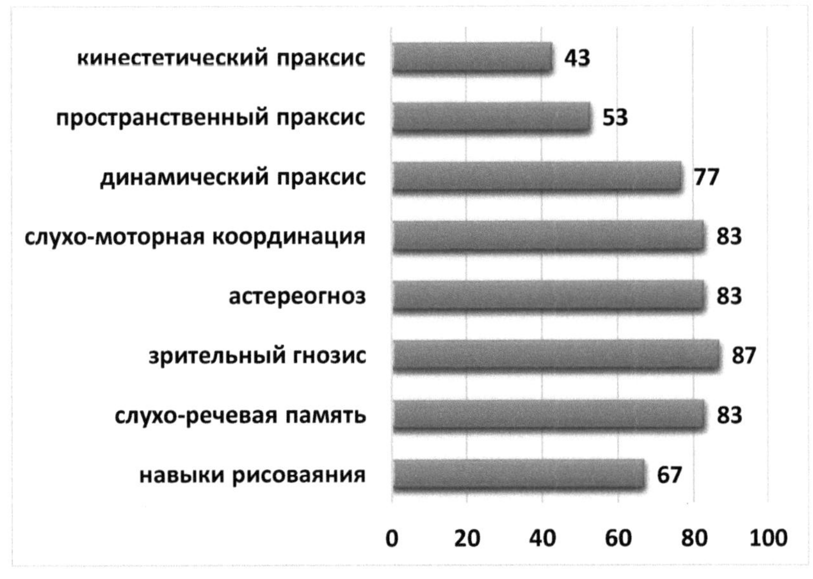

Figure 3.4. Cognitive disorders in the studied children with autism

Drawing impairment and auditory-verbal memory impairment occurred about equally in both groups (67% and 83% in the main group and 57% and 77% in the comparison group, respectively).

Conclusions of the chapter

The prevalence of medium and high risk of RAS development according to the M-CHAT-R screening questionnaire (45 and 40%, respectively) has been established among the examined children. Criteria for early diagnosis of RAS in children based on the analysis of the M-CHAT-R screening scale and DSM V criteria were developed.

Neurological symptomatology in children with autism depends on age and is characterized by the presence of diffuse microsymptomatology in the form of dissociation of tone, changes in reflexes (mild asymmetry of tendon and periosteal reflexes), low speech production and the presence of a defect in social communication. Changes in the neurological status of patients with early infantile autism are most often characterized by changes in tendon reflexes, muscle tone, and lesions of the hMN.

Neurologic syndromes (pyramidal, extrapyramidal insufficiency syndrome, muscular dystonia syndrome, enuresis and others) may be the result of a fairly high frequency of subclinical forms of central nervous system damage in the perinatal period.

CHAPTER 4. RESULTS OF THE ANALYSIS OF NEUROPROTEIN CONTENT AND ELEMENTAL COMPOSITION OF HAIR

4.1 Microelement composition of hair in children with autism spectrum disorders

Micronutrients play a significant role in the functioning of the nervous system. Experimental and clinical data have been accumulated indicating that the reason for the development of pathological symptoms and diseases (including diseases of the nervous system) may be the unbalanced content of macro- and micronutrients in the human body. Nowadays, people are exposed to significant exposure to toxic substances, which significantly affects their health [12, 123]. The imbalance of essential and toxic substances in the human body can cause the growth of all kinds of diseases, including autism spectrum disorders (ASD).

Despite the significant genetic component in determining the risk of RAS development, most cases are multifactorial in nature and are realized with the participation of certain pathogenetic factors [38, 56]. Such factors include immune disorders, oxidative imbalance, exposure of the organism to toxic agents and insufficient intake of essential nutrients [48, 92].

Due to the multifactorial nature of most cases of RAS, the question arises about the relevance of identifying specific risk factors for a particular territory of residence, population, ethnic group.

This chapter presents the peculiarities of micronutrient composition of hair of children with RAS. Sixty-one children with ASD were examined. It is generally believed that the composition of elements in hair reflects their intake over a long period of time (months, years), whereas fluctuations in the level of bioelements, short-term in terms of exposure and significant in terms of intake, are more rapidly reflected in fluids, including blood [68].

Twenty-four elements in the hair of children with RAS were studied. The obtained data are presented in Table 4.1.

Average content of trace elements in the hair of children with ASD

(µg/g)

Elements	Averages	Mean deviation	Reference values
Na	1124,992	156,299	250-800
Cl	6138,016	554,424	1000-2000
Ca	339,836	20,334	1000-1500
Sc	0,004	0,0001	0,006-0,015
Cr	0,381	0,091	0,35-1,0
Mn	0,538	0,074	0,35-1,0
Fe	19,121	1,151	20-30
Co	0,039	0,007	0,05-0,1
Cu	7,626	0,669	15-20
Zn	108,369	7,771	150-250
K	1330,656	189,955	800-1000
Se	0,418	0,011	0,35-1,0
Br	177,126	55,956	1-3,2
Rb	0,933	0,126	0,5-1,0
Ag	0,203	0,053	0,1-0,25
Sb	0,082	0,025	>0,2
I	0,778	0,209	0,8-1,5
La	0,025	0,008	0,02-0,04
Au	0,015	0,003	0,02-0,05
Hg	0,041	0,013	0,1-0,3
U	0,121	0,026	0,1-0,3
As	0,108	0,007	0,1-0,3
Ba	1,600	0,180	1,0-5,0

As can be seen from the presented data in children with RAS there is a significant increase in sodium (1124,99±156,3 µg/g with reference values of 250-800 µg/g), chlorine (6138,0±554,4 µg/g with reference values of 1000-2000 µg/g), potassium (1330,7±189,9 µg/g with reference values of 800-1000 µg/g), bromine (177,1±55,9 µg/g with reference values of 1,-3,2 µg/g) and decrease of such parameters as calcium (339,8±20,3 µg/g with reference values of 1000-1500 µg/g), zinc (108,4±7,8 µg/g with reference values of 150-250 µg/g) and iron (19,1±1,2 µg/g with reference values of 20-30 µg/g).

The study of the content of macronutrients showed that in children with RAS in 47.5% of cases there is an increase in the level of sodium, in 83.6% - chlorine against the background of a decrease in calcium in 100% of cases, and in 80.3% of cases of normal values of potassium (Fig. 4.1).

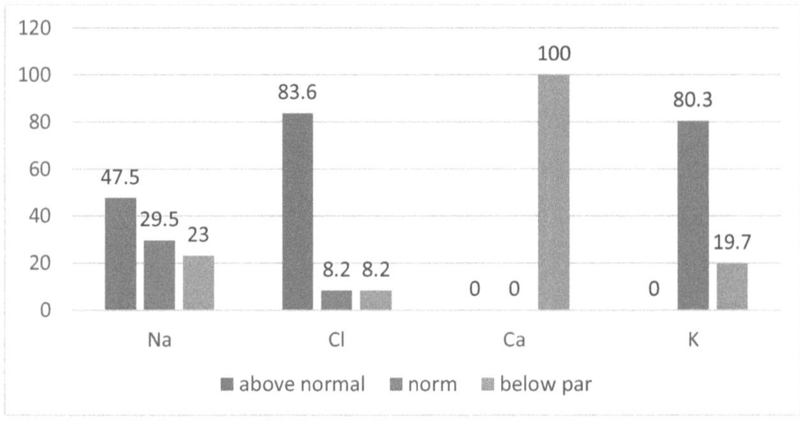

Figure 4.1. Analysis of macronutrient content in hair of children with RAS

Among essential trace elements in children with RAS, there is a decrease in copper in 95.1% of cases, cobalt in 82.0%, chromium in 80.3%, zinc in 77.0%, and iodine in 75.4%. These essential elements decrease

against the background of increased bromine in 86.9% and normative values
of selenium in 80.3% and manganese in 63.9% (Fig. 4.2).

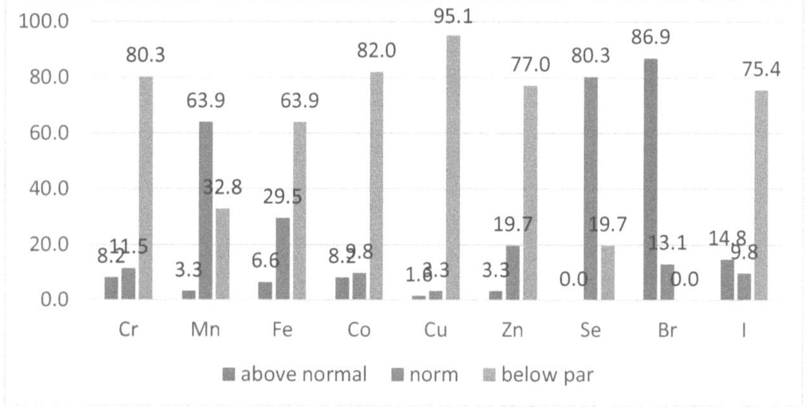

**Figure 4.2. Analysis of the content of essential trace elements in
hair of children with RAS**

Reduced zinc and copper, may play a role in the GABA system, which
is likely altered in autistic syndrome.

In children with RAS, a deficiency of macronutrients and vital
elements such as iron, zinc, manganese, selenium and cobalt has been
identified, the level of which is significant for epigenetic regulation of the
genome, and disorders at the epigenetic level are considered as possible
causes of neurodevelopmental disorders leading to autism spectrum
disorders [9].

As can be seen from Diagram 4.3, children with RAS have low content
of toxic trace elements in most cases, however, it should be noted that 31.1%
have high levels of rubidium and 21.3% have high levels of silver.

Complex excess of toxic micronutrients, leads to disruption of
important metabolic and respiratory processes by substitution of essential
micronutrients and, as a consequence, may increase the risk of developing
RAS.

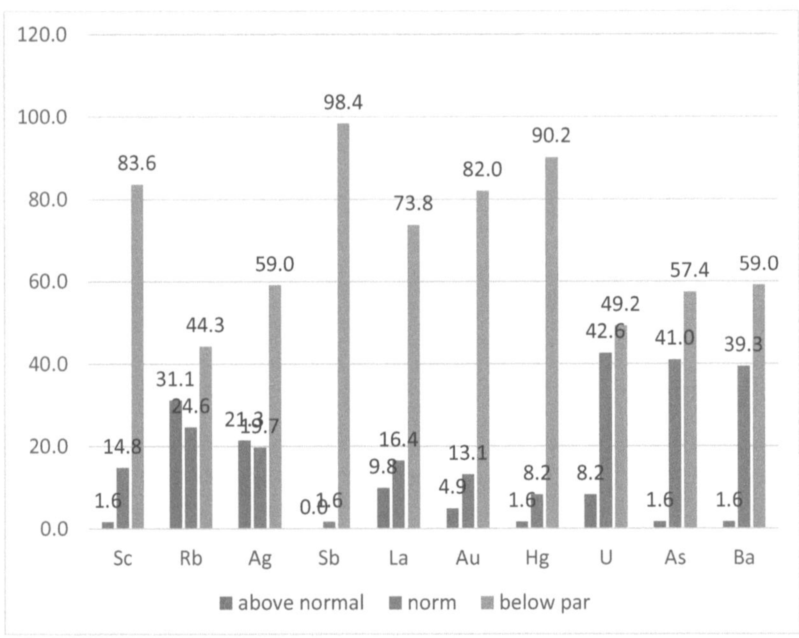

Figure 4.3. Analysis of the content of toxic trace elements in hair of children with RAS

Children with RAS who have an excess of toxic metals have a higher ATEC test score (60 points or more), which supports the assumption that high levels of toxic metals are important for the risk of developing this condition.

We have established a correlation between macro and microelement status and the severity of RAS in children (Fig. 4.4).

Thus, the highest direct correlations were obtained with sodium, chlorine and bromine, i.e. the higher the content of these macronutrients, the more severe the degree of RAS. Inverse high and average correlation with essential trace elements such as calcium, chromium, iron, cobalt, copper, zinc, iodine was also established.

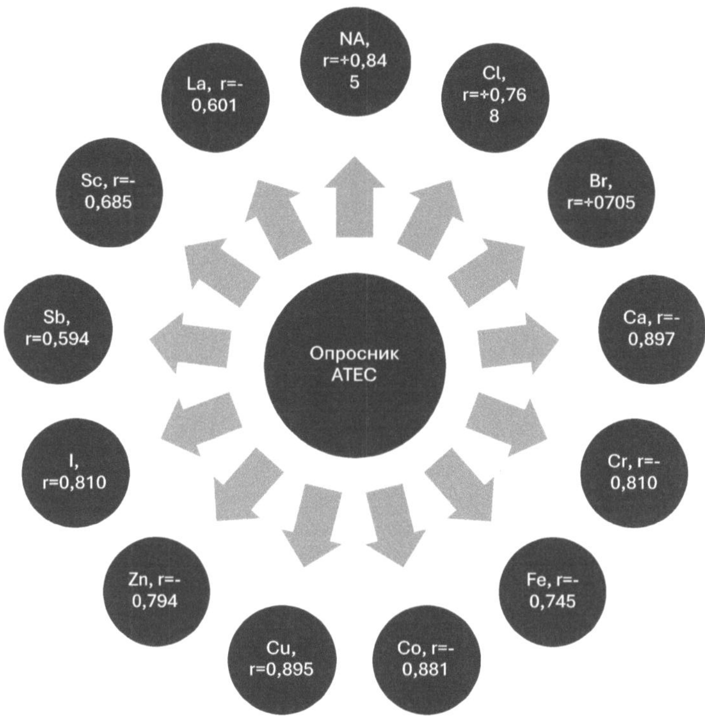

Fig. 4.4. Indicators of correlation between macro and microelemental hair stotav and severity of RAS according to the ATES questionnaire

Considering that all studied toxic trace elements in our study were lower than normal, however, we found their influence on the development of RAS, which was proved by high inverse relationship in correlation analysis.

4.2 Neuroimmunologic indicators of children with autism spectrum disorders

Various neurochemical systems (glutamatergic, GABAergic, serotoninergic, dopaminergic, etc.) play an important role in the activity and maturation of the central nervous system.

The fact that these systems interact at the receptor level during CNS development is particularly important for understanding brain functioning in norm and pathology. This makes it necessary to clarify and, possibly, revise the existing hypotheses of the pathogenesis of neuropsychiatric diseases in children, in particular, RAS in children.

When assessing the average content of S100B protein in the serum of OG children, its significant increase was observed in comparison with that of CG children (p=0.005) (Fig. 4.5).

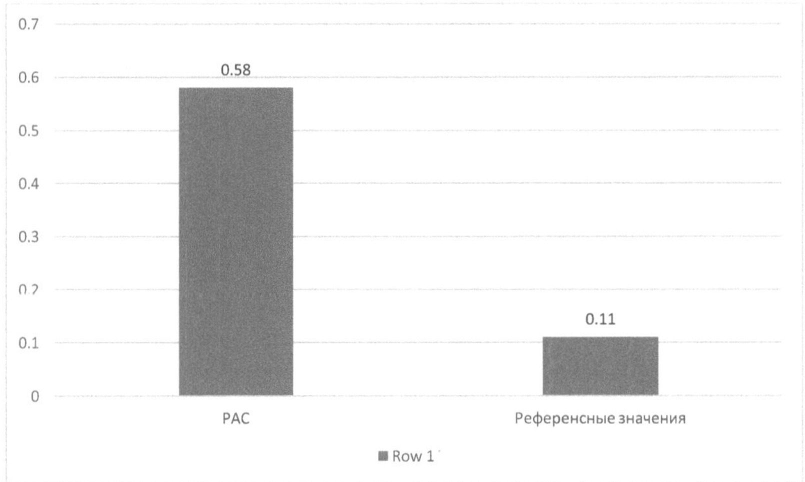

Figure 4.5. S100B content in children with RAS

Fourteen (31%) children with RAS had S100B scores slightly above or at the upper limit of normal in contrast to the CG children.

In severe course of RAS, S100B indices were high, and in moderate severity of the disorders there was a difference from the indices in the control group. The majority of children with RAS have signs of stressed neuroprotective mechanisms, and children with abnormalities of brain structures development have signs of hypoxic-ischemic brain damage.

Neuron-specific enolase is one of the structural varieties of the enolase enzyme, which is required for glycolysis and is therefore present in all cells of the body. The isoforms of this enzyme are tissue specific. Neuron-specific enolase, NSE, an isoform specific to neurons, is characterized by some structural features necessary for the normal functioning of this enzyme at elevated chloride ion concentrations.

In addition to the cytoplasm of neurons, NSE is also found in cells of neuroendocrine origin, such as chromaffin cells of the adrenal medulla, parafollicular cells of the thyroid gland, and some others. However, increased synthesis of this enzyme occurs in tumor cells, which ensures a high rate of glycolysis, active tumor growth and its spread to surrounding tissues.

Elevated NSE is often seen in small cell lung cancer, as well as in medullary thyroid cancer, pheochromocytoma, neuroendocrine tumors of the intestine and pancreas, and neuroblastoma.

Children with RAS showed a 12.4-fold increase in NSE relative to normative values (5.46±0.84 versus 0.44±0.03; P<0.001) (Figure 4.6).

The appearance of reduced serum levels of antibodies to OBM indicates a disruption of the blood-brain barrier, most significant in patients with RAS.

At the same time, partial or complete loss of myelin by viable outgrowths can lead to pronounced disturbances in the conduction of nerve impulses.

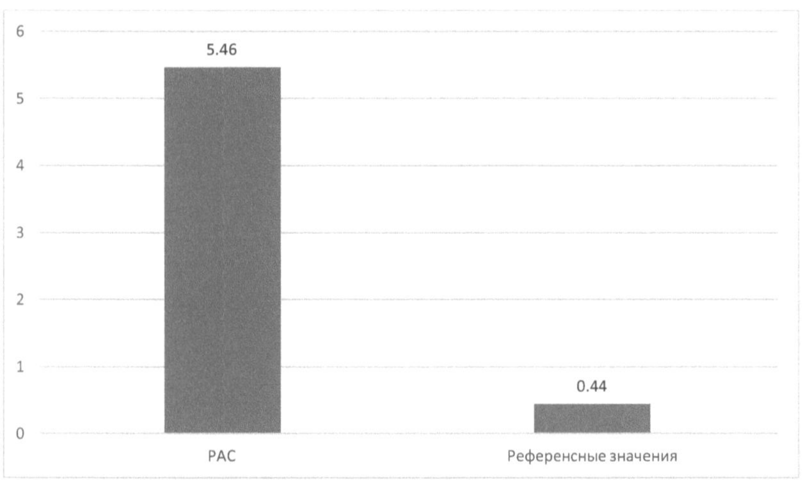

Figure 4.6. NSE-IFA-BEST scores in children with RAS

Demyelination of the axon significantly reduces the speed of conduction of nerve impulses, so that the conduction process will no longer be salticatory between Ranvier intercepts, as in a myelinated fiber, and the movement of electrolytes (K^+ and Na^+) will occur across the entire axon surface. This may lead to the formation of new ion channels in the cell membrane and increase the concentration of potassium ions in the extracellular space, which in turn may alter nerve cell excitability and exacerbate paroxysmal brain activity.

Children with RAS showed an almost 2-fold decrease in MVR relative to controls (0.69±0.02 versus 0.35±0.03; P<0.05) (Figure 4.7).

It should be noted that GFAP plays a fundamental role in maintaining the normal functioning of both individual astrocytes and the CNS as a whole. Changes in its content have important clinical significance in diseases of the nervous system.

In the mature CNS, this neurospecific protein is found in protoplasmic gray matter astrocytes, fibrous white matter astrocytes and plays an important role in their differentiation.

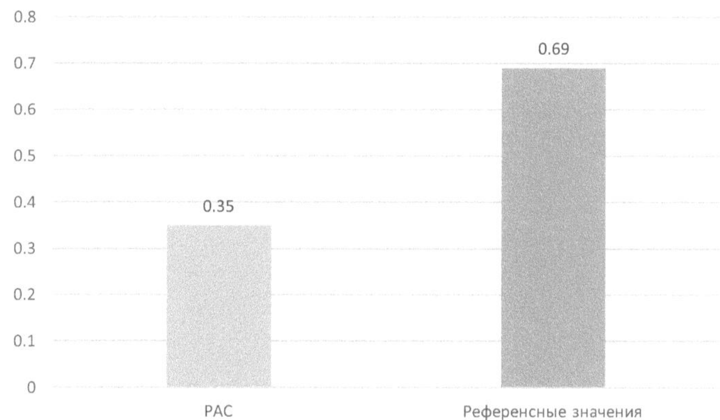

Figure 4.7. MBP-Myelin Basic Protein scores in children with RAS

Near the surface of the brain, GFAP is concentrated in astrocytes forming the superficial boundary glial membrane (membrane limitans gliae superficialis), and is found in large amounts in subependymal astrocytes near the ventricles of the brain.

The results obtained by V.A. Berezin (2010) indicate that there is a correlation between the degree of impaired GEB permeability and the amount of GFAP penetrating into the blood. Thus, the presence of AAT to GFAP in serum also indirectly indicates a violation of the barrier function of the GEF in the examined children with RAS (Fig. 4.8).

As can be seen from the presented data, there was an increase in GFAP scores 12.3 times relative to normative values (0.37±0.008 versus 0.03±0.002; P<0.001).

Serotonin has many functions in the body, including mood, sleep, appetite and sociality. In the gastrointestinal tract it stimulates the muscles involved in digestion, in the circulatory system it causes blood vessels to constrict or dilate, and in the brain it transmits messages between neurons. Its concentration in the brain is closely linked to depression.

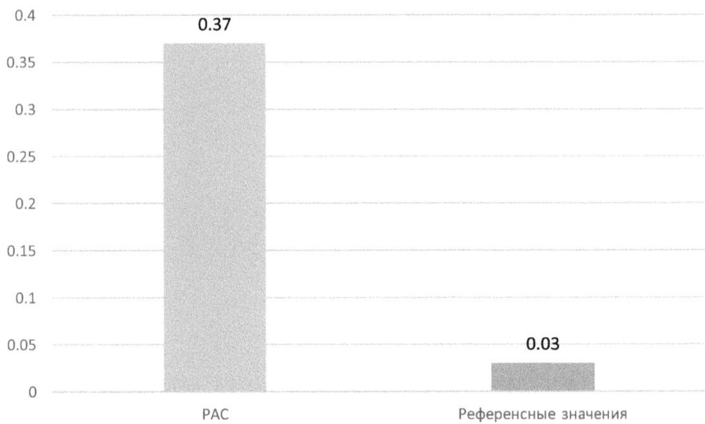

Figure 4.8. GFAP scores in children with RAS

Children with RAS were found to have an almost 3-fold increase in blood serotonin, which on average reached 3.45±0.07, whereas in the control group it was 1.05±0.08 (P<0.01) (Figure 4.9)

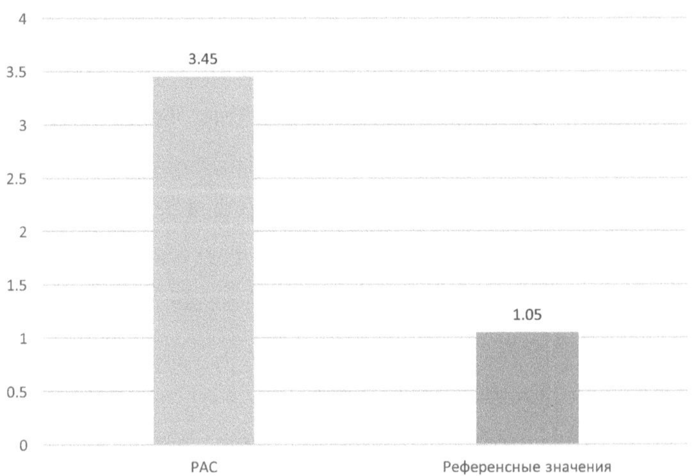

Figure 4.9. ST-Serotonin values in children with RAS

Thus, in children with RAS there is an imbalance in the neuroimmunologic status, so there is an increase in the level of S100B, NSE, GFAP against the background of a decrease in OBM and ST-Serotonin.

Conclusions of the chapter

In hair samples of children with RAS, a decrease in the level of macronutrients (sodium, chromium and bromine), essential elements (calcium, chromium, zinc, copper, iron, cobalt, iodine) involved in the functioning of the nervous and immune systems was found.

A tendency to increase the content of toxic trace elements (rubidium, silver, lanthanum, uranium) was found. The correlation between the level of macronutrients, essential elements and increased scores in the ATES test reflecting the clinical status of children with autism spectrum disorders has been established.

Almost 12-fold increase of NSE and GFAP level, 5-fold increase of S100B level in relation to the normative values against the background of 2-fold decrease of OPM and 3-fold decrease of serotonin were found. S100B is known to modulate specific binding activity of acetylcholine, γ-aminobutyric acid, norepinephrine, dopamine and serotonin receptors. In addition, it participates in the implementation of genetic programs of apoptosis and antiapoptotic protection, and together with GFAP is the main component of reparative processes occurring in the brain after various kinds of damage.

High values of NSE, GFAP and S100B indicate impaired proliferation of glial cells and maturation of brain neurons and contribute to the realization of neurodegenerative action. Children with RAS have high levels of serotonin, almost 3-fold increase in relation to reference values

CHAPTER 5. EVALUATION OF THE EFFECTIVENESS OF MICROCURRENT REFLEXOTHERAPY IN AUTISM

To analyze the results of the study on the effectiveness of the MTRT method, we divided children with autism into two groups. The main group consisted of 80 children with autism who received MTRT sessions in complex pharmacological treatment and ABA therapy.

MERT was performed using the "MERT" device authorized for use in the European Union (registration number MED 31494_1). During MERT, ultra-small electrical signals were used, which are applied to various biologically active points to restore the patient's own normal brain and spinal cord function. The full course of treatment is 3 weeks - 15 therapeutic procedures. Treatment is carried out daily, the duration of a treatment procedure varies from 30 minutes to 40 minutes.

The comparison group consisted of 40 children with autism receiving standard pharmacotherapy and ABA therapy.

As a result of the conducted studies, an improvement was found, which had in some cases a reliable character, but for all developmental indicators of children with RAS there was a tendency to improvement in the main group in relation to the comparison group.

In the comparison group, all indicators of children's development showed positive dynamics in the course of treatment, but the reliability was registered only for the indicator "Absence of the pronoun "I" in the lexicon".

The inclusion of MTRT in the complex treatment promotes the recovery of a child with RAS not only developmental skills, but also the leveling of symptoms of anxiety and phobias - almost 2 times, in relation to the comparison group, where children received only pharmacotherapy.

As a result of the studies, improvement was found to be significant in some cases, but for all developmental indicators of children with RAS, there was a trend towards improvement in the main group in relation to the comparison group (Figure 5.1).

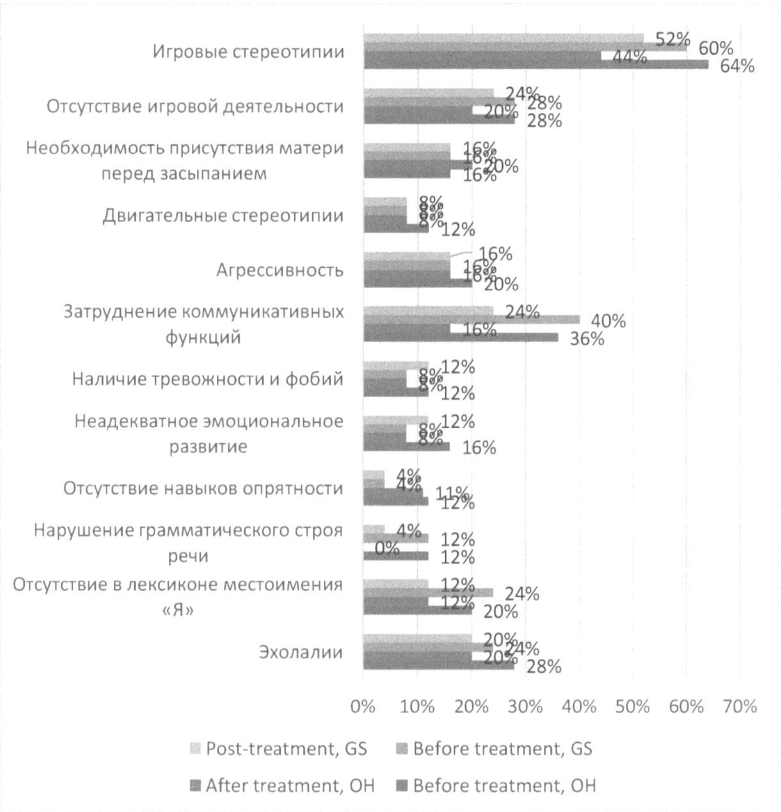

Fig. 5.1. **Development of examined children with RAS in the dynamics of therapy**

In addition, we conducted research to study the dynamics of visual and auditory-verbal memory, attention, thought processes, and emotional sphere (Table 5.1).

Table 5.1.

Examination data of children with DA before and after

71

treatment

Indicators	Main group		Comparison group	
	Before treatment	After treatment	Before treatment	After treatment
Data on the dynamics of visual and auditory-verbal memory indices				
Visual memory capacity (first presentation)	1.5 figures	2.9 figures	1.24 figures	1.7 figures
Auditory-verbal memory capacity (first presentation)	2.1 words.	3.75 words.	2.2 words.	3.0 words.
Data on the dynamics of attention indicators				
Number of errors per 1 min	9,1	7,3	8,8	8,1
Data on the dynamics of indicators of thinking productivity				
Number of completed tasks	2,05	4,1*	2,3	3,4
Data on the dynamics of emotional sphere indicators				
Phobias	6,1	2,7*	6,9	4,9
Anxiety	7,3	3,6*	6,4	4,2
Aggressive reactions	7,6	3,3*	7,7	6,1
Depressive reactions	5,4	1,9*	5,8	4,2

Note: * - reliability of data before and after treatment (P<0.05)

As can be seen from the data presented in the table, in children with RAS with the inclusion of RTT there is a recovery of visual and auditory memory indicators in the dynamics of treatment, but the figures were not reliable, but had a more pronounced trend in relation to the comparison group.

A similar picture is observed when analyzing the attention indicators in the dynamics of treatment, in the main group children made errors 1.5

times less often, while in the comparison group - 1.1 times. According to the data obtained, the reliability of the data was not significant, but had a pronounced trend in the main group of children with RAS.

When administering MTRT in complex treatment, children in the main group showed a 2-fold increase in productive attention, whereas in the comparison group 1.5 times (P<0.05).

In the emotional sphere there was also a significant leveling of indicators in children with RAS in the main group in relation to the data before and after treatment, as well as to the indicators of children from the main group (P<0.05)

By the end of the treatment positive dynamics was noted: cognitive interest to the surrounding increased, fatigue, excitability, manifestations of aggressiveness decreased.

The volume of working memory in the visual modality increased 1.93 times; in the auditory-verbal modality - 1.76 times. Arbitrary attention became more stable, the number of errors decreased by 1.28 times.

After the past course of treatment, the child was able to complete an average of 2.95 more tasks, thinking productivity increased 3.57 times.

After the course of treatment, phobias became less, anxiety decreased, aggressive and depressive reactions also decreased.

In 52% of cases, children of the main group showed positive dynamics of cognitive activity of moderate and expressed degree; 40% of children showed weakly positive dynamics and only 8% of children showed no dynamics. 8% of children had positive dynamics of a pronounced degree, these children showed a significant improvement in emotional state, the emergence of arbitrary activity, a decrease in motor stereotypes, and the emergence of communicative speech function.

In children treated according to the standard methodology, positive dynamics of a pronounced degree was noted in only 8%, cognitive dynamics of a moderate degree in 28% of children, in 36% - a weak degree, in 28% of cases there was no dynamics, i.e. no dynamics and weak dynamics in 64% of cases; only 36% of children had moderate and pronounced dynamics.

The mean score on the ATES - test in the main group decreased from 61.94 to 42.21 points (almost 20 points), while in the comparison group, this index decreased from 61.86 points to 48.1 points (about 14 points).

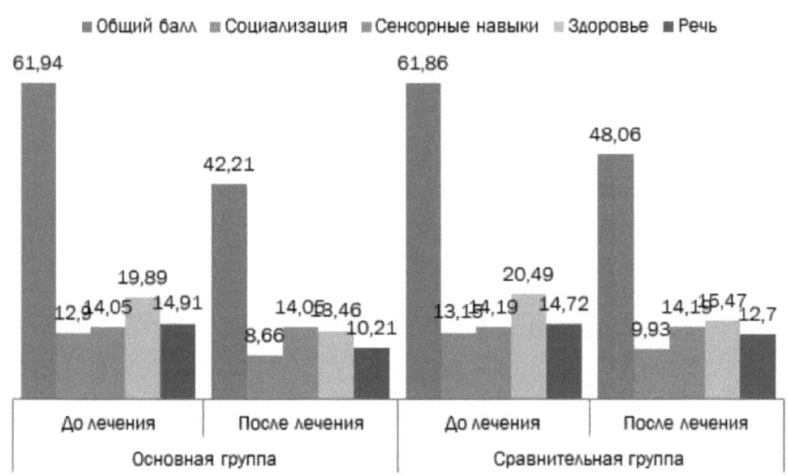

Figure 5.2. **Assessment of treatment efficacy by the ATEC test (scores)**

This trend was also observed in the other subscales, which indicates the effectiveness of RTT for children with ASD

In 52% of children with RAS in the main group there is a pronounced positive dynamics in the cognitive sphere, whereas in the comparison group only 8% of children managed to achieve a pronounced positive dynamics, which was significant (Fig. 5.3).

Weak positive dynamics was observed in 40% of children in the main group and in 64% of children in the comparison group. The absence of dynamics of cognitive activity was observed 3.5 times less often in children in the main group and 28% in the comparison group.

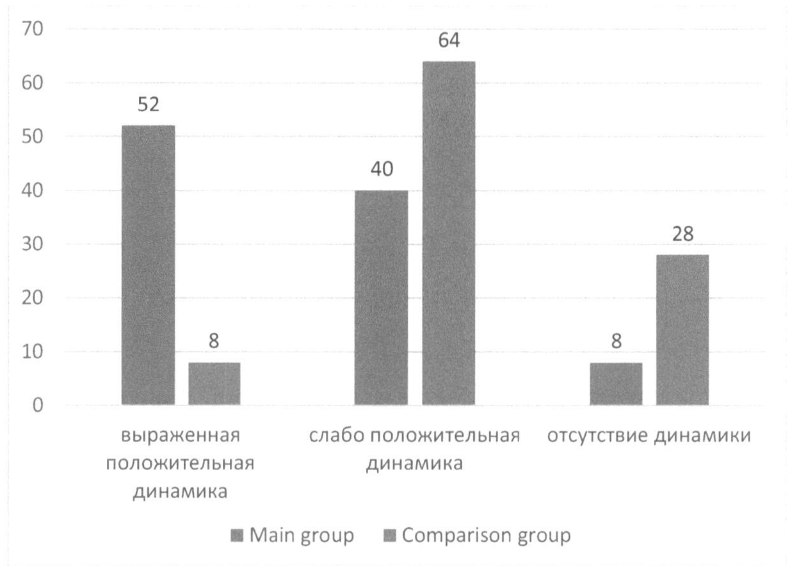

Fig. 5.3. Dynamics of cognitive activity in the process of treatment of children with RAS

Conclusions of the chapter:

Significantly significant improvements in social adaptation and increased sociability in patients with early infantile autism were found after the inclusion of RTT in the treatment complex.

In children with RAS, who received MTRT in the complex treatment increased speech skills, attention productivity, visual modality, decreased anxiety, aggression and depressive reactions, as well as the acquisition of communication skills by an average of 45.3%.

CONCLUSIONS.

1.   Early diagnosis of RAS should be made with the inclusion of the DSM5 criteria together with the M-CHAT screening method, which will make it possible to assess the severity of neurological and psycho-emotional defects and reflect the state of the child's socio-communicative status. Among 405 children with complaints of lack of sociability, speech, presence of stereotyped, repetitive behavior, limited interests and hobbies according to the screening questionnaire M-CHAT-R a prevalence of medium and high risk of RAS development was found (45 and 40% respectively).

2.   As a result of the developed criteria for early diagnosis of RAS based on the analysis of the M-CHAT-R screening scale and DSM V criteria, 29.6% of children were diagnosed with RAS.

3.   Children with RAS have an imbalance of neuroprotein content in the blood, which is characterized by a significantly significant increase in the level of S100B (5.3-fold; $P<0.001$), NSE (12.4-fold; $P<0.001$), GFAP (12.3-fold; $P<0.001$) and ST-Serotonin (3-fold; $P<0.01$) against the background of decreased OPM (2-fold; $P<0.05$). Based on cross-correlation analysis, the influence of neuroprotein imbalance on the development of RAS severity in children was proved.

4.   Analysis of macronutrients and trace elements in the hair composition of children with RAS showed a decrease in the level of macronutrients (calcium), essential elements (chromium, zinc, copper, iron, cobalt, iodine) involved in the functioning of the nervous and immune systems. A tendency to increase the content of toxic trace elements (rubidium, silver, lanthanum, uranium) has been found. The correlation between the level of macronutrients, essential elements and increased scores in the ATES test reflecting the clinical status of children with autism spectrum disorders has been established.

5.   Complex medication neuroprotective treatment of RAS in children in combination with non-medication methods - MTRT led to significant improvements in speech and social interaction skills, as well as the acquisition of communication skills by an average of 45.3%.

<h1 align="center">PRACTICAL RECOMMENDATIONS</h1>

1.   The complex of multilevel diagnostics in patients with early infantile autism including clinical and neurological, neuropsychological, use of special scales, and in particular M-CHAT-R, allowing to determine the functional state of the central nervous system, is offered;

2.   Children of preschool age should be under continuous dynamic observation until school age for the purpose of early diagnosis and timely correction of detected disorders.

3.   The study of neuroimmunologic indices should be included in the complex of diagnostic measures in the early diagnosis and differential diagnosis of RAS.

4.   The use of MTRT should be included in the complex of therapeutic measures for psycho-speech correction of patients with RAS.

REFERENCE LIST

1. Barylnik Y.B., Aleshina N.V. Pathogenic factors in the history of children, preceding the formation of symptoms of early childhood autism (organic and procedural) //Vestnik neurology, psychiatry and neurosurgery. 2013. № 6. C. 18-22.

2. Protein s100b and autoantibodies to it in the diagnosis of brain damage in craniocerebral injuries in children/E. G. Sorokina, J. B. Semenova, O. K. Granström, et al. G. Sorokina, J. B. Semenova, O. K. Granström, et al //Journal of Neurology and Psychiatry. C.C. Korsakov. - 2010. - T. 110. № 8. - C. 30-35.

3. Protein s100v in the blood of children with autism spectrum disorders/T. F. Golubova, L. A.. Tsukurova, L. L. Korsunskaya and others //Journal of Neurology and Psychiatry. C.C. Korsakov. - 2019. - T. 119. № 12. - C. 76-83.

4. Bobylova M.Y., Vinyarskaya I.V., Bystrova K.Y., Narovatkina Y.K. Atypical autism in children: features of somatoneurological status and outpatient observation by a general pediatrician // Russian Journal of Pediatric Neurology. 2013. T. 8. № 4. C. 42-51.

5. Bobylova M.Yu., Mironov M.B., Kulikov A.V., Kazakova M.V., Bogacheva M.A., Tankevich Y.A., Glukhova L.Y., Barletova E.I., Abramov M.O., Mukhin K.Yu, Rudenskaya G.E. Clinical case of SYNGAP1 gene mutation, C2214_2217DELTGAG DE NOVO in a girl with epilepsy, mental retardation, autism and motor disorders // Neurology, Neuropsychiatry, Psychosomatics. 2014. № 2. C. 34-40.

6. Variation in the content of satellite 3 (1q12) in the genomes of blood leukocytes of mentally healthy children and children with autism/S. G. Nikitina, Y. M. Chudakova, G. V. Shmarina, et al: Psychiatric science in history and perspective. Proceedings of the Jubilee All-Russian Scientific and Practical Conference with international participation, dedicated to the

75th anniversary of the Scientific Center of Mental Health. - 2019. - C. 212-213.

7. Vinarskaya A. Kh. Calcium-binding protein s100b and some problems of neurology/A. Kh. Vinarskaya, T. Kh. Bogodvid, V. V. Andrianov// Eurasian Scientific Association. - 2020. - № 4-3 (62). - C. 146-150.

8. Influence of bischofite baths on the indicators of S100B protein in blood plasma in children with autism spectrum disorders : scientific edition / T. F. Golubova [et al.] // Vestnik rehabilitativnaya meditsina : Association of specialists of rehabilitative medicine; Union of rehabilitation specialists of Russia. - 2020. - N 4. - C. 48-54

9. Voronkova K.V., Pylaeva O.A., Kholin A.A. Epilepsy and autism.// Vestn Epileptologii 2012;(1):12-20.

10. Serum glutamate in autism and other disorders of psycho-verbal development in children / T. A. Mityukova, T. V. Dokukina, O. E. Polulyakh, et al. A. Mityukova, T. V. Dokukina, O. E. Polulyakh and others //Laboratory Diagnostics. Eastern Europe. - 2020. - T. 9. № 4. - C. 420-430.

11. Glukhova L.Y. Autistic epileptic regression. // Vestn Epileptologii 2012;(1):3-12.

12. Golubova T.F., Tsukurova T.F., Nuvoli A.V., Vlasenko S.V., Savchuk E.A. effect of bischofite baths on the indicators of S100B protein in plasma in children with autism spectrum disorders. vestnik regenerative medicine. 2020; 98 (4): 48-54. https://doi.org/10.38025/ 2078–1962–2020–98–4–48–54

13. GC-enriched fragments of extracellular DNA induce apoptosis in peripheral blood lymphocytes of children with autism/Yu.M. Chudakova, E.S. Ershova, N.N. Veiko et al: Proceedings of the XXIII Congress of the I. P. Pavlov Physiological Society with international participation. - 2017. - C. 373-375.

14. Zavadenko N.N., Pechatnikova N.L., Simashkova N.V., Zavadenko A.N., Orlova K.A.Neurological disorders in children with autism// Russian journal of perinatology and pediatrics. 2015. T. 60. № 2. C. 14-21

15. Ivanov, M.V. Results of epidemiological screening of the risk of autism spectrum disorders in young children / M.V. Ivanov, N.V. Simashkova, G.V. Kozlovskaya // Bulletin of the Council of Young Scientists and Specialists of the Chelyabinsk region. 2016. T. 3. № 2 (13). C. 56-59.

16. Karashchuk L.N., Razzhivina M.I. The problem of autism in the modern world // Person in a changing world: health, adaptation, development. 2014. № 1 (4). C. 29-35.

17. Korovina N. Yu. Biochemical blood analysis as one of the methods in the diagnosis of autism / N. Yu. Y. Korovina, D. I. Zolatorev, T. T. Batysheva / / Child and Adolescent Rehabilitation. - 2019. - № 4 (40). - C. 37.

18. Kosarev M. O. Changes in neuron-specific enolase (nse) and protein s100 in serum of patients with dyscirculatory encephalopathy with concomitant anxiety disorders/M. O.. O. Kosarev: Collection of scientific papers of young scientists dedicated to the Day of Russian Science . - 2018. - C. 74-78.

19. Kotlyarov V.L. Motor stereotypes in the structure of psychotic and non-psychotic autism spectrum disorders / V.L. Kotlyarov, N.V. Simashkova, G.V. Kozlovskaya, M.A. Kalinina, M.V. Ivanov // Mental Health. 2016. T. 14. № 2 (117). C. 69-78.

20. Leshchenko, S. V. Autism in children: causes, types, signs and recommendations to parents // Young Scientist. - 2018. - № 48 (234). - C. 253-257.

21. Maltsev D. V. Expanded clinical and laboratory phenotype in genetically determined folate cycle disorder in children with autism spectrum disorders // International Journal of Neuroscience. - 2018. - №. 5 (99).

22. Misyuk N.N. Neurophysiological studies in autism / N.N. Misyuk, T.V. Dokukina, S.A. Marchuk, N.A. Sergeeva, S.A. Greben // Psychiatry, Psychotherapy and Clinical Psychology. 2012. № 4 (10). C. 96-109.

23. Mukhin K.Y. Cognitive epileptiform disintegration and similar syndromes. In: Mukhin K.Y., Petrukhin A.S., Kholin A.A. Epileptic encephalopathies and similar syndromes in children. Moscow: Art-Service Ltd, 2011. C. 396-426.

24. Nikolskaya O. S., Baenskaya E. R., Liebling M. M. Autistic child / Nikolskaya O. S., Baenskaya E. S., Baenskaya E. R., Liebling M. M. M.: Terevinf, 2017, 134 p.

25. Nikolskaya O.S. Structure of mental health disorders in pediatric autism. Almanac of the Institute of Correctional Pedagogy of the Russian Academy of Education. 2014. № 18-1. C. 3.

26. Nikolskaya O.S., Baenskaya E.R., Liebling M.M. Autistic child. Ways of help. Moscow: Terevinf, 2010, 288 c.

27. Nogovitsyn V.Y., Nesterovsky Y.E., Osipova G.N. et al. Epileptiform activity in children without epilepsy: clinical-electroencephalographic correlations. //Jurn Neurol Psychiatr 2013;(6):42-6.

28. Prognostic value of the determination of maternal autoantibodies in the period of pregravidar preparation, affecting the development of autism spectrum disorder in the child : scientific edition / A. M. Torchinov [et al.] // Obstetrics and Gynecology. - M., 2017. - N12. - C. 60-66.

29. Proteomic analysis of the protein profile of blood sera of children with autism/A. L. Kaisheva, A. T. Kopylov, I. Yu Yurov, S. G. Vorsanova, et al. L. Kaisheva, A. T. Kopylov, I. Yu Yurov, S. G. Vorsanova et al //Voprosy prakticheskaya pediatria. - 2016. - T. 11. № 5. - C. 12-17.

30. Rabbani N. Autism spectrum disorders: in search of blood biomarkers. Rabbani, P. D. Thornalley// Autism and developmental disorders. - 2019. - T. 17. № 1 (62). - C. 15-23.

31. Rostomashvili I.E., Ufaeva N.Yu. The peculiarity of the manifestation of communication in preschoolers with early childhood autism and its development by means of hippotherapy // Uspekhi sovremennoi nauki. 2016. T. 6. № 10. C. 129-135.

32. Simashkova N.V. Atypical autism in childhood. Avtoref. dis. ... Dr. of medical sciences. 2013. 44 c.

33. Simashkova N.V. New approaches to the problem of atypical autism. In: Proceedings of the XIV Congress of Psychiatrists of Russia. M., 2016. C. 223.

34. Simashkova N.V. Effective pharmacotherapy and rehabilitation of patients with autism spectrum disorders. Journal of Neurology and Psychiatry. C.C. Korsakov. 2011. № 3. C. 14.

35. Simashkova N.V., Klyushnik T.P., Koval-Zaitsev A.A., Yakupova L.P. Clinical and biological approaches to the diagnosis of pediatric autism and childhood schizophrenia // Autism and developmental disorders. 2016. T. 14. № 4 (53). C. 51-67.

36. Simashkova NV, Yakupova LP, Bashina VM Clinical and neurophysiologic aspects of severe forms of autism in children // Zhurn neuropathol psychiatr 2013;106(7):12-9.

37. Strozenko L. A. et al. Distribution of folate cycle genes in the population of adolescents in Barnaul, Altai Krai // Mother and Child in Kuzbass. - 2015. - №. 1.

38. Tatarkova E. A. et al. Influence of polymorphic variants of folate cycle genes on the process of early termination of pregnancy in the residents of the Republic of Adygea //Vestnik Adygeya State University. Series 4: Natural-mathematical and technical sciences. - 2016. - №. 1 (176).

39. Trailin A. V. V. Protein s100v: neurobiology, significance in neurological and psychiatric pathology/A. V. Trailin, O. A. Levada//International Neurological Journal. - 2009. - № 1. - C. 166-175.

40. Thrombodynamic indices of blood hypercoagulability in children with infantile autism and pediatric schizophrenia/ O. S. Brusov. S. Brusov, N. V. Simashkova, N. S. Karpova, M. I. Factor, S. G. Nikitina // Journal of Neurology and Psychiatry. C. C. Korsakov. - 2019. - T. 119. № 1. - C. 59-63.

41. Thrombodynamic indicators of hypercoagulability with spontaneous clots in plasma and pediatric autism: correlation relationship with severity of catatonia/O. S. Brusov, N. V. Simashkova, N. S. Karpova, et al: Psychiatric Science in History and Perspective. Proceedings of the Jubilee All-Russian Scientific and Practical Conference with international participation, dedicated to the 75th anniversary of the Scientific Center of Mental Health. - 2019. - C. 175-178.

42. Platelets as a model of neurons in biochemical studies in psychiatric diseases/I. S. Boksha, O. K. Savushkina, T. A. Prokhorova, et al. S. Boksha, O. K. Savushkina, T. A. Prokhorova, et al //Medico Pharmaceutical Journal Pulse. - 2022. - T. 24. № 1. - C. 15-24.

43. Filippova N. V., Barylnik Y. B. Epidemiology of autism: a modern view of the problem // Social and Clinical Psychiatry. 2014. T. 24, № 3. C. 96-101.

44. Khalimova H. M. Extrapyramidal casalliclard s100v oksil mikdorining xarakatga boglik boulmagan belgilar bilan uzaro boglikligi / H. M. Khalimova, R. J. Matmurodov / Journal of Theoretical and Clinical Medicine. M. Khalimova, R. J. Matmurodov/Journal of Theorietical and Clinical Medicine. - 2016. - № 2. - C. 91-94.

45. Chigrinets A.N. Concept, signs of early childhood autism and strategies to support children with early childhood autism // Lomonosov Readings in Altai: fundamental problems of science and education: Collection of scientific articles of the international conference. Altai State University. 2015.C. 2248-2249.

46. Abrahams B.S., Geschwind D.H.. Connecting genes to brain in the autism spectrum disorders. Arch Neurol 2010;67(4):395-9.

47. Ajabi, Samereh, Farhad Mashayekhi, and Elham Bidabadi. "A study of MTRR 66A> G gene polymorphism in patients with autism from northern

48. Boddaert N., Zilbovicius M., Philipe A. et al. MRI findings in 77 children with nonsyndromic autistic disorder. PLoS One 2009;4(2):e4415.

49. Bosco, Paolo, Rosa-Maria Guéant-Rodriguez, Guido Anello, Concetta Barone, Farès Namour, Filippo Caraci, Antonino Romano, Corrado Romano, and Jean-Louis Guéant. "Methionine synthase (MTR) 2756 (A→G) polymorphism, double heterozygosity methionine synthase 2756 AG/methionine synthase reductase (MTRR) 66 AG, and elevated homocysteinemia are three risk factors for having a child with Down syndrome." American Journal of Medical Genetics Part A 121.3 (2014): 219-224.

50. Bottema-Beutel K, Malloy C, Lloyd BP, Louick R, Joffe-Nelson L, et al. Sequential Associations Between Caregiver Talk and Child Play in Autism Spectrum Disorder and Typical Development.Child Dev. 2017 May 26.

51. Brian JA, Smith IM, Zwaigenbaum L, Bryson SE.Cross-site randomized control trial of the Social ABCs caregiver-mediated intervention for toddlers with autism spectrum disorder.Autism Res. 2017 Jun 2.

52. Brown AC, Crewther DP.Autistic Children Show a Surprising Relationship between Global Visual Perception, Non-Verbal Intelligence and Visual Parvocellular Function, Not Seen in Typically Developing Children.Front Hum Neurosci. 2017 May 11;11:239.

53. Buie T., Campbell D.B., Fuchs G.J. 3rd et al. Evaluation, diagnosis, and treatment of gastrointestinal disorders in individuals with ASDs: a consensus report Pediatrics 2010;125 Suppl 1:S1-18.

54. Coutinho E, Jacobson L, Pedersen MG, Benros ME, Nørgaard-Pedersen B, et al. CASPR2 autoantibodies are raised during pregnancy in mothers of children with mental retardation and disorders of psychological development but not autism.J Neurol Neurosurg Psychiatry. 2017 Jun 1. pii: jnnp-2016-315251.

55. Demirci E.Autism Spectrum Disorder and Phenylketonuria: Dyzygotic Twins with Double Syndrome. Noro Psikiyatr Ars. 2017 Mar;54(1):92-93.

56. Deonna T., Roulet-Perez E. Epilepsy and autistic disorders. In: Trimble M., Schmitz B. et al. The neuropsychiatry of epilepsy. 2nd ed. Cambridge University Press, 2011. P. 24-38.

57. Ecker C, Schmeisser MJ, Loth E, Murphy DG.Neuroanatomy and Neuropathology of Autism Spectrum Disorder in Humans.Adv Anat Anat Embryol Cell Biol. 2017;224:27-48.

58. Emanuele E., Orsi P., Boso M. et al. Low-grade endotoxemia in patients with severe autism. Neurosci Lett 2010;471(3):162-5.

59. Freitag C.M., Staal W., Klauck S.M. et al. Genetics of autistic disorders: review and clinical implications. Eur Child Adolesc Psychiatry 2010;19(3):169-78.

60. Gepner B., Feron F. Autism: a world changing too fast for a mis-wired brain? Neurosci Biobehav Rev 2009;33(8):1227-42.

61. Hudac CM, Stessman HAF, DesChamps TD, Kresse A, Faja S, et al. Exploring the heterogeneity of neural social indices for genetically distinct etiologies of autism.J Neurodev Disord. 2017 May 26;9:24.

62. James, S. Jill, Stepan Melnyk, Stefanie Jernigan, Oleksandra Pavliv, Timothy Trusty, Sara Lehman, Lisa Seidel, David W. Gaylor, and Mario A. Cleves "A functional polymorphism in the reduced folate carrier gene and DNA hypomethylation in mothers of children with autism. Cleves, "A functional polymorphism in the reduced folate carrier gene and DNA hypomethylation in mothers of children with autism." American Journal

of Medical Genetics Part B: Neuropsychiatric Genetics 153.6 (2010): 1209-1220.

63. Kalb LG, Stuart EA, Mandell DS, Olfson M, Vasa RA.Management of Mental Health Crises Among Youths With and Without ASD: A National Survey of Child Psychiatrists.Psychiatr Serv. 2017 Jun 1:appips201600332.

64. Kamp-Becker I, Poustka L, Bachmann C, Ehrlich S, Hoffmann F, et al.Study protocol of the ASD-Net, the German research consortium for the study of Autism Spectrum Disorder across the lifespan: from a better etiological understanding, through valid diagnosis, to more effective health care.BMC Psychiatry. 2017 Jun 2;17(1):206.

65. Kathuria A, Sala C, Verpelli C, Price J.Modelling Autistic Neurons with Induced Pluripotent Stem Cells.Adv Anat Anat Embryol Cell Biol. 2017;224:49-64.

66. Khetrapal N. The framework for disturbed affective consciousness in autism. Neuropsychiatr Dis and Treat 2017;4(3):531-3.

67. Koegel RL, Oliver K, Koegel LK.The Impact of Prior Activity History on the Influence of Restricted Repetitive Behaviors on Socialization for Children With High-Functioning Autism.Behav Modif. 2017 Jun 1:145445517706346.

68. Kogan M.D., Blumberg S.J., Schieve L.A. Prevalence of parent-reported diagnosis of autism spectrum disorder among children in the US, 2017. Pediatrics 2009;124(5):1395–403.

TABLE OF CONTENTS

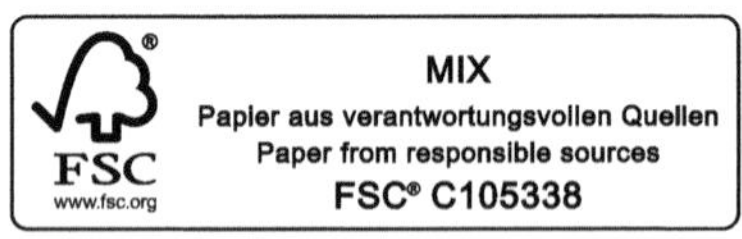